Strategies
for Teaching Nursing

Strategies for Teaching Nursing

SECOND EDITION

Rheba de Tornyay, R.N., Ed.D., F.A.A.N.
Professor and Dean
School of Nursing
University of Washington
Seattle, Washington

Martha A. Thompson, R.N., M.S.N., M.A.Ed.
Associate Professor
Department of Nursing
San Jose State University
San Jose, California

1807 1982

A Wiley Medical Publication
JOHN WILEY & SONS
New York • Chichester • Brisbane • Toronto • Singapore

Library of Congress Cataloging in Publication Data:

de Tornyay, Rheba.
　　Strategies for teaching nursing.

　　(A Wiley medical publication)
　　Bibliography: p.
　　Include index.
　　1.　Nursing—Study and teaching.　I.　Thompson,
Martha A.　II.　Title.　III.　Series.

RT71.D38 1982　　　610.73′0711　　　82-2786
ISBN 0-471-04523-3　　　　　　　　　　AACR2

Printed in the United States of America

10 9 8 7 6 5 4 3 2 1

To Our Families

Preface

It has been more than a decade since the first edition of *Strategies for Teaching Nursing* was published. During this time new instructional technologies have appeared and are available to the nursing instructor. A major change in the second edition is the inclusion of teaching strategies designed to help nursing students to be self-directing, help them learn at their own pace, and individualize learning. However, nursing instructors still use traditional approaches when teaching groups of students. We hope that this book will help nursing instructors to consider new approaches as well as improve old methods in teaching.

This book is divided into three parts. The first part discusses the components of teaching, which were originally designed for practice in a microteaching laboratory. These components were selected from those identified by the Stanford Teacher Education Program (1967) study and later adapted for use at the University of California, San Francisco, School of Nursing (de Tornyay & Searight, 1968). These components help the teacher to become sensitized to some of the essential acts performed as an instructor. Regardless of what is taught or where, the teacher is a reinforcer of desired behaviors in students, uses examples and models to explain concepts, seeks simulated work situations, and helps students to develop the psychomotor skills needed to practice nursing. Teachers ask questions to stimulate students, as well as to find out if they understand what has been taught, to motivate students toward learning through the use of set induction, and to help toward closure for a class, unit of work, course, or the entire nursing program.

The second part discusses the skillful combining of teaching components into three old, but still sound, teaching strategies. Lecturing remains a major teaching strategy for exposing large numbers of students in our nursing programs to the major concepts needed for practice. We believe that there is a legitimate reason for lecturing and hope that this chapter will help the nursing instructor to deliver a lecture with organization, clarity, and purpose. The seminar, or discussion, method is also a prevalent strategy used by teachers of nursing in both the classroom for theory development and the pre- and postclinical conferences with nursing students. To provide students with the opportunity to be exposed to faculty members with varying clinical backgrounds and to allow instructors of nursing to teach within their own specialty areas in the generalized undergraduate nursing program, team teaching is frequently used as a teaching strategy. We have included sections on the major advantages and disadvantages for each of the three group teaching strategies discussed.

The third part discusses the major strategies used to individualize learning. The first chapter in Part 3 includes a description of the characteristics necessary to consider instruction to be individualized. The remaining chapters discuss three innovations in educational technology that are useful for achieving this goal.

The learning module is fast becoming a standard in nursing education. It is a currently available strategy that can be used to increase the extent to which instruction in nursing is individualized. Chapter 12 provides guidelines for developing and using learning modules in nursing education. Learning contracts also offer a readily available option to those nursing instructors who want to focus on individualized learning. The elements of learning contracts are discussed, and a sample from a nursing situation is included. Computer-assisted instruction (CAI) is one strategy that is not, at present, used in most nursing education settings. In the belief that one of the reasons for this is that nursing faculties are unfamiliar with CAI, this chapter explores the types and uses of CAI as an introduction to those without prior computer experience. It is hoped that interest in using the computer for educational purposes will increase and that teachers of nursing will become aware of the computer's potential for helping achieve individualized instruction.

None of the methods discussed in Part 3 is seen as a panacea for all of nursing education; however, we do believe that nursing educators should make use of available technology for improvement of their teaching and, thus, the learning of students.

We hope that this book will be a helpful guide for many teachers of nursing. It is written not only with the new teacher in mind; we believe that it will be useful for the experienced teacher as well. As the knowledge base for nursing has expanded tremendously in the past few years, graduate programs in nursing have tended to decrease preparation in the "functional area" of teaching. Therefore, the teacher of nursing may well enter a teaching career with neither the prerequisite trial of competence nor experience with the tools for teaching. When teachers have limited preparation for teaching, they tend to teach as they were taught. It is our hope that this book will expand the horizons for teachers of nursing by offering alternatives and options to strengthen the teaching–learning process.

We hope that we do not sound prescriptive in our approach to teaching. The selection of a teaching strategy is dependent on many factors. First, the objectives to be achieved must be considered. Objectives provide the basis for the selection of appropriate learning experiences and instructional strategies. When students know precisely what the objectives are (because they have been formulated in terms of descriptions of minimum performance requirements), they have direction for their activities, and the learning process has more relevance. Mager (1962) points out that if the learner is given a copy of the instructional objectives, the teacher may have to do little else! We believe this viewpoint is a bit extreme, and it is toward the "something else" that this book is written.

Second, planning for teaching involves consideration of the kind of material to be taught and learned. For example, in teaching students to understand physiological changes resulting from specific pathological problems, an expository, or telling, approach may be desirable because the subject matter is fairly stable. Also, students will have difficulty understanding major concepts if they do not have an adequate background of facts and generalizations. However, in helping students to understand how various patients and clients deal with loss, the teacher may wish to use a more experiential approach in order to help students toward a greater understanding of the concept.

The teaching strategy to be selected involves a third and most important consideration. Each teacher is different and brings his or her own unique style and personality to the teaching–learning process. Effective teachers make use of a number of teaching techniques. They have their own individual teaching styles because they know that they cannot perform successfully when they are not comfortable with themselves and with what they are doing; but, effective teachers also realize that it becomes boring to both themselves and their students when their range of activities is unnecessarily limited. They are willing to try new ways of helping their students learn. They know that teaching and learning should be exciting, fun, and stimulating. We hope that our book will help teachers of nursing to see new ways to help their students achieve the learning objectives.

The underlying assumption for this book is that teaching skills can be learned. We do not accept the old adage that "teachers are born, not made." We also believe that teaching, to be effective, cannot be based solely on a "bag of tricks." Teaching skills are performance behaviors and such skills have rational reasons for being selected. We have attempted to include the learning principles relevant to each of the teaching techniques we describe and hope that our book will help to bridge the gap between theory and practice.

This book is intended to be only one educational resource for the teacher of nursing. It is meant to supplement texts on educational psychology, instructional objectives, approaches to clinical teaching in the health sciences, and evaluation of learning. Therefore, we wish to emphasize that this small book was not intended to be complete in itself.

Rheba de Tornyay
Martha A. Thompson

Acknowledgments

We wish to thank the following people for their input and helpful reviews of chapters during the work on this second edition: Juliet Corbin, Joan Perry, Kathy Rose-Grippa, Leslie Strayer, Toni Taylor, and Lucille Whaley. Their suggestions helped greatly to improve the end result presented. Our appreciation is extended to Mary DeMeneses for her willingness to share her experiences with us in the use of learning contracts in graduate education. We are grateful to Sharon Eaton and Grace Davis for their contribution. We thank Vicki Carney for her capable help in preparing the manuscript.

Rheba de Tornyay
Martha A. Thompson

Contents

PART 1

THE COMPONENTS OF INSTRUCTION

1

Employing Reinforcement

Reinforcement is a major condition for most learning. It is among the most powerful procedures used in teaching. Reinforcement techniques can be varied to provide different effects depending on the types of learning we want students to acquire. Because of its importance we have chosen to consider this component before the others.

As a learning theory, reinforcement has its root in Thorndike's *Law of Effect*. From his studies dealing with cats, rats, and humans, Thorndike formulated general laws from his laboratory data. The *Law of Effect* (Thorndike, 1911) states:

> Of several responses made to the same situation, those which are accompanied or closely followed by satisfaction will, other things being equal, be more firmly connected with the situation so that when it recurs, they will be more likely to recur; those which are accompanied or closely followed by discomfort will, other things being equal, have their connections with that situation weakened, so that when it recurs, they will be less likely to recur.

Stimulus-response (S-R) learning theory explains behavior in terms of the association between stimulus and response. Learning is represented in terms of the systematic changes in S-R associations. The term reinforcement is used to refer to the events that strengthen responses.

DEFINITION OF REINFORCER

A *reinforcer* is anything that strengthens behavior and increases the probability of its recurrence. There are, of course, both positive and negative reinforcers. In the teaching-learning process, Skinner (1953) views positive and negative reinforcers as incentives for students. Put in its most simple terms, a positive reinforcer is a positive reward. A negative reinforcer is a negative reward—a stimulus that gives relief from something unpleasant. Examples of positive reinforcement include praise, smiles, money, prizes, being recognized, doing a task well, and other pleasurable responses from others. Examples of negative reinforcement include relief from pain or discomfort. A student will learn to make a response that will enable her or him to escape an uncomfortable situation.

EFFECTS OF POSITIVE REINFORCEMENT

In employing reinforcement, the teacher, of course, must know what behaviors are to be reinforced. Is it the correct answer? Is it thinking through a difficult problem, even when the answer is only partially acceptable? Is it participating in a classroom discussion? Is it performing a task smoothly? Is it being willing to tackle a difficult task? Is it being willing to try again after making a mistake? Is it being willing to share one's own ideas? Is it being willing to share one's own feelings?

The literature abounds with examples of the effects of positive reinforcement. In a study (Verplanck, 1955) designed to test the influence of reinforcement on students' verbalization of opinions, each time a student began a statement with such phrases as "I think . . ." or "I believe . . ." or "It seems to me that . . . ," the experimenters used such reinforcers as "You're right" or "I agree with you" or rephrased the student's statement. They nodded, smiled, and utilized other nonverbal positive reinforcers to indicate their approval. When reinforced in this way, the students tended to volunteer their opinions more readily. When the reinforcers were withdrawn by the experimenters by ignoring the remarks of the students, or by such statements as "I certainly disagree with that," the number of opinion statements made by the students sharply decreased.

Anderson, White, and Wash (1966) were interested in determining whether praised students would perform better than reproved students. Further, they wished to test the hypothesis that school achievement was a critical variable in the effects of praise and reproof. They tested the following two hypotheses:

H_1 Praised students will perform better than reproved students.

H_2 Reproved low achievers and praised high achievers will perform better than praised low achievers and reproved high achievers.

The subjects for their study were university students in a course in educational psychology. An objective test of the subject matter was utilized as the criterion test. In addition, an objective test in mathematics was used to determine if behaviors would be transferred to a different subject area. Results indicated that there was greater achievement increment in performance in both subject areas when praise was used rather than reproof with both the low achieving student and the high achieving student. Their findings lend support to the notion that praise may assist in the transfer of learning from one area to another.

The previous two studies were selected to illustrate one of Hilgard's (1956, p. 486) principles of learning: learning under the control of reward is usually preferable to learning under the control of punishment; and learning motivated by success is preferable to learning motivated by failure.

Let us now turn to some of the ways in which positive reinforcement is employed. The more obvious verbal ways are by saying "good" or "fine" or "yes" when a student responds. The more obvious nonverbal ways are by nodding, smiling, moving toward the student, and generally looking pleased. Additional reinforcing behaviors include calling the student by name, writing the student's comments on the chalkboard, or repeating comments and referring back to what a student has contributed. Statements such as "That indicates careful thinking on your part," "Your comments showed good grasp of principles," "It is apparent that you have included information gained from your other courses," and "I like the initiative you showed in your nursing care today" not only act as positive reinforcers for students, but also indicate the kind of behavior the teaching is rewarding. Teachers sometimes comment that the student has displayed creativity or originality in a term paper and yet fail to be specific about the reasons for reaching that conclusion. When a student solves a problem in an inventive way, a comment telling how the actions show originality helps to guide this behavior for the future and fosters repetition.

A very powerful reinforcing behavior is a request from the teacher for a student to share successful experience with others. For example, telling a student "I am impressed with the nursing care you gave today in working with a patient demonstrating multiple nursing care problems and hope that you will share your care plan with others" gives the student recognition and prestige with classmates. It is, of course, essential to recognize the achievements of each student in the group rather than always turning to the better student, as tempting as it may be.

A very major problem for every instructor is determining what, in fact, constitutes positive reinforcement for an individual student. Reinforcement can be highly personal. A reinforcer for one student may affect another student quite differently. We know that individual differences in people mean that rewards to the individual are closely tied to their own value system. Whereas praise, recognition, and encouragement are universally valued, the quantity of reinforcement is an unknown factor for effectiveness with each individual student. Mild praise can be strongly reinforcing to a student whose failures may have been outnumbering successes, while high praise may be relatively ineffective for the student who consistently achieves honors. Another factor to consider is that the effects of many events are transitory. A reinforcer for a given student at one time may not be the one for another time. Glaser (1969) makes the point that when attempts are made by teachers to allow students more participation in decision making, it may be initially reinforcing for students to receive more power to act on their own. But later many may feel that they do not want to make decisions and the effect loses its power.

CLASSIFICATION OF REINFORCERS

Tosti and Addison (1979) have attempted to classify educational reinforcement in a systematic way in order to help teachers identify what may serve as a reinforcer for some students, at least some of the time. Although their list appears to be most applicable for classroom teachers in grades 1–12, the general categories could well be applied to college classes in nursing. Their taxonomy includes the following:

I. *Recognition*
Praise
Certification of accomplishments
Formal acknowledgements (awards, testimonials, letters of recommendation)
Informal acknowledgements (private conversations, "pat" on back)
Publicity (note in school newspaper, public press)

II. *Tangible rewards*
Grades
Food (free lunch)
Prizes

III. *Learning activities*
Opportunity for desirable enrichment assignment ("honors" class)
More interesting, or more difficult clinical assignments

IV. *School responsibilities*
Opportunity for increased self-management

Opportunity for more frequent or more participation in decision making

Acceptance of suggestions for improving curriculum

Greater opportunity to select own goals for learning experiences

Greater opportunity to control own schedule and set own priorities

V. *Status indicators*

Appointment as a peer tutor

Having own space (study, carrel, desk)

VI. *Incentive feedback*

Increased knowledge of examination scores

Knowledge of individual contributions (helping others)

VII. *Personal activities*

Opportunity to engage in special projects

Extra time off

It is important to point out that reinforcers will motivate students only if they are contingent upon learning performance. The reinforcer must be the result of, or must be directly linked to, student accomplishments. Tosti and Addison (1979) aptly point out that the indiscriminate use of reinforcers may result in happy students but may not result in *productive* students. Again, it is exceedingly important that the instructor constantly keep the instructional objectives in mind in determining what to reinforce.

It is relatively easy for teachers to practice giving positive reinforcement when students are correct. But what should be done about a wrong response? Obviously, teachers do not wish to reinforce an incorrect answer. The way in which students are told that they are wrong is important here. Ignoring the response really doesn't tell what the error is; rather, it leaves students wondering whether they are right, partially right, or what. When teachers say, "No, that's really not it," they let students know they are not on the right track. It is possible to reward students for trying, as well as let them know that they are not right. In other words, it is possible to be accepting of the person while rejecting the idea or response presented.

EFFECTS OF NEGATIVE REINFORCEMENT

Essentially, a negative reinforcement is punishment. Skinner (1953) escribes punishment as the removal of a positive reinforcer and the a dition or substitution of an aversive stimulus. When an individual student is ignored or ridiculed in any way, the teacher's behavior serves as negative reinforcement. We have all observed classrooms where the students are reluctant to volunteer ideas or responses. This occurs when individual students have experienced embarrassment, rejection, or have failed to be heard. Not only will the embarrassed student be reluctant to participate again, but other students tend to withdraw in the fear that the same treatment will be forthcoming to them.

Mager (1968) makes an eloquent case for what he terms positives and aversives in developing attitudes toward learning. Following his list of what he terms "universal aversives," every nurse can probably trace reactions to specific clinical areas or nursing care problems to the way she or he was introduced to material or taught in the courses that related to these areas. Painful learning occurs when cramped into small working quarters or having to hold instruments until one's wrists hurt. Confusion happens when excessive noise is present or when directions cannot be heard. Fear and anxiety occur when, by word or deed, students are told that it is doubtful if their actions will lead to success or that the grades will reflect the fact that almost no student is superior. Frustration is common when too much information is given too rapidly or too soon to be absorbed by the learner. Students are made to feel insignificant when the teacher ignores a student's question. Teaching one thing and testing another leads to dejection among students. The list goes on and on and is, indeed, a sad commentary on the educational process.

There is no question but that the conditions of punishment and reward are not clear-cut or unambiguous for adult learners. There is some evidence (Solomon, 1964) that if an individual receives some aversive stimulation along with positive reinforcement, the punishment procedure may actually strengthen the positive response. This is most clearly demonstrated by the methods employed by some stop smoking clinics, in which a mild electric shock treatment is administered preceding any positive comments to deter the clients from smoking. Be that as it may, it is highly unlikely that any nursing instructor should involve such drastic techniques to foster learning!

POSSIBLE REASONS FOR FAILURE TO USE POSITIVE REINFORCEMENT

Given the fact that there is overwhelming evidence supporting the generalization that reinforced responses tend to be repeated in given situations, whereas nonreinforced responses tend to be discontinued (De Cecco & Crawford, 1974), it is interesting to speculate on the reasons why nursing instructors too often fail to reinforce desired behaviors. Possibly it may be linked to the prevalent notion that praise will spoil a child, and this notion carries forward to the adult learner. It must be fresh in the memory of any nurse that when the instructor did *not* say something it meant everything was all right. As nursing instructors, we are quicker to point out what improvement a student needs rather than reinforce the worthy behavior. Somehow, we expect the student to experience intrinsic motivation, and we are overconvinced at times that the student really does not need to be told when doing well. One might wonder how many nursing students have changed majors because of inadequate support in terms of positive reinforcement during the early nursing experiences. Nursing is difficult enough to master, and the novice nurse cannot help but feel inadequate (one might add parenthetically, the same goes for the experienced nurse!) much of the time.

KNOWLEDGE OF RESULTS AS REINFORCER

A very major reinforcing event for a student is knowledge of results. In practicing motor skills, knowledge of results assists in improving the skill. Nursing students frequently find out if they have performed a nursing procedure correctly by the results achieved. For example, if the student neglects to replace fluid with air while withdrawing fluid from a sealed vial by means of a syringe, the student soon learns by the difficulty in withdrawing the fluid that the pressure within the vial has been reduced. This example illustrates one of Hilgard's (1956, p. 487) learning principles. He points out that information about the nature of good performance, knowledge of one's own mistakes, and knowledge of successful results aid learning. Practice is valuable to the student only when there is knowledge of results.

This idea of knowledge of results has implications when we provide students with information about the correct answers following a written examination. Many years ago, the effect of grading examinations was studied in high school science courses (Curtis & Woods, 1929). Tests consisting of 100 objective-type items were administered to a large number of high school students. The teachers followed four different procedures in returning the tests, as follows:

1. Teacher read the correct answer while each student corrected his own paper. Discussion followed.
2. Teacher marked wrong responses, but wrote nothing else on the paper. Papers were returned and discussed item by item.

3. Teacher wrote in all corrections, and papers were returned and treated as in Number 2 above.
4. Teacher wrote in all corrections, but when papers were returned only specific questions asked by students were discussed.

The test was repeated the next day and 6 weeks later to determine short-term and longer-term retention. A consistent pattern of merit for the four methods was demonstrated. Number 1 was most effective; Numbers 2 and 3 were equal; and Number 4 was poorest.

Whereas this last example illustrates the effect of immediate feedback for a content-oriented approach, it is possible that immediate feedback may be contraindicated for some teaching strategies.

In the learning and problem-solving divisions described by Bruner (1966), the problem-solving cycle is called trial-and-error, means-end testing, trial-and-check, hypothesis testing, and many others. The problem-solving cycle involves the formulation of a test of trial, the operation of the testing procedure, and the comparison of the results of the test with some criterion. Bruner carefully points out that knowledge of results is useful, depending on when the learner receives the corrective information. For example, if knowledge of results occurs too early in the problem-solving sequence, it may be ineffective, either because the learner cannot understand the implications of the feedback information, or because it actually interferes with learning for oneself.

Timing for knowledge of results feedback may be important. Sullivan, Schutz, and Baker (1971) found that immediate knowledge of results of a multiple choice item was more effective than a delayed-feedback procedure when given to ROTC cadets in a university program. Their study gives credence to the effects of letting students score their own classroom tests in order for the knowledge of results to be provided immediately.

Knowledge of the importance of supplying feedback has provided the impetus for the technological innovations in instruction that will be discussed in Part 3. There is no question that programmed instruction and computer-assisted instruction aid learning, not only by allowing the student to progress at an individual rate, but because of its ability to provide immediate feedback through the knowledge of results of actions.

GRADES AS REINFORCERS

Whereas grades are considered one of our most important motivational devices (McKeachie, 1963), there appears to be an incredible lack of research on the effect of grading on student learnings. We all know that grades are important to students. We know for certain that most students are motivated to get sufficiently high grades to remain in college. The nursing student who aspires to graduate school is motivated to get grades high enough to unlock the door to further education. Grades can bring about the kind of learning the instructor desires. If teachers base their grades on memorization of details, then students will memorize the text to receive the positive reinforcement of a good grade. If students are rewarded for integrating and applying principles, then they will try to acquire such ability. Grades can be utilized as an incentive for learning, as they can provide positive reinforcement for students. Using grades chiefly as a threat may produce avoidance through negative reinforcement.

PROVIDING CONDITIONS TO FOSTER POSITIVE REINFORCEMENT

One way of providing positive reinforcement is by seeking experiences for students so that they will succeed. The old adage of "nothing succeeds like success" is really helpful. By providing instruction in increments we can allow for success most of the time. We do not simply place students in situations we know they cannot handle. We build up to the more difficult nursing situations, if that is at all possible. We recognize that students were not ready to tackle a given nursing situation if they find themselves in one, and we help them with their problem-solving techniques so that they learn how to cope with the problem themselves. We give the student some control over the selection and sequencing of the instruction. Probably most important of all is when we can express genuine delight in the student's success. The idea to be conveyed by the teacher is "I know you can do it," rather than "prove to me that you can achieve."

Brodie (1969) carefully points out that there may be a difference of perception between student and teacher. Students may interpret lack of response from the instructor as negative reinforcement. They may express inability to please the teacher no matter what is attempted. The teacher, on the other hand, may actually have thought that the student was doing a good job and failure to comment may have meant there was no criticism. Therefore, it is important to remember that the lack of a positive response is, in fact, negative reinforcement.

The instructor who provides experiences with a prediction of success for the student helps the student store a backlog of success that can compensate for later failures and thus provide a tolerance for failure. The very nature of nursing practice is such that we hardly have to go out of our way to seek experiences that will cause feelings of inadequacy for the nursing student. These occur regularly enough in the day-to-day nursing experiences. By helping students to accentuate the positive, we help them cope with their failures in a constructive way.

The very essence of the power of positive reinforcement has been stated simply and eloquently by Jackson (1966):

> . . . offering appropriate praise, not just because positive reinforcers strengthen response tendencies, but because the student's performance is deserving of human admiration. It means responding *as* an individual *to* an individual.

GROUP REWARD STRUCTURE

We have focused on individual rewards in this chapter. However, in nursing, as in other professions, effective performance frequently requires the cooperative performance of a group of professionals. The effects of cooperative, competitive, and individual reward structures on performance have been systematically studied during the past 50 years, unfortunately, not with uniform results. Slavin and Tanner (1979) define a reward structure as a set of rules under which rewards are distributed to individuals contingent upon their performance. A *cooperative* reward structure is one in which individuals depend on one another's performance to be rewarded, as in a collaborative project. A *competitive* reward structure is one in which one person's success requires another's failure, such as in competitive sports. An *individual* reward structure is one in which the connection between a person's behavior and the earned rewards does not depend on any other person's performance.

Because it is important to help nursing students toward the goal of cooperation, nursing faculty should seriously consider rewarding students for cooperative behaviors. Slavin and Tanner (1979) found in their study, which was designed to investigate the conditions under which a cooperative reward structure increased productivity and learning more than an individual structure, that students in the cooperative reward structure groups performed at a higher level in terms of initial learning and retention than did the students in the individual reward groups. The study focused on reading comprehension as one of the traditional learning tasks in high school and, hence, may not be directly transferable to the learning tasks of nursing. Nevertheless, it behooves every nursing instructor to develop some learning activities in which the entire group is rewarded for the activity, if cooperative behavior as a learning objective is to be rewarded.

There is still another factor that bears emphasis. Research evidence clearly supports the conclusion that cooperative reward structures are much more positively associated with "social connectedness" (Slavin, 1977). This is a term that social scientists use to describe the degree to which an individual feels attracted to others and feels and acts a part of a valued group. These social dimensions include interpersonal attraction, friendliness, positive group evaluation, helpfulness, and other positive feelings towards colleagues. That these attributes are important to foster in the neophyte nurse is not open to question. However, that these behaviors are not always developed is clearly observable when one observes the overt and covert behaviors and attitudes of some nurses at work and the attitudes of coworkers to one another. Increases in mutual attraction as a consequence of a cooperative reward structure have been obtained by a number of investigators in studies that have employed different group sizes, tasks, ages, and durations, yet the finding of greater interpersonal attraction occurring with a cooperation rather than a competitive structure has persisted (Slavin, 1977). Abundant evidence exists reinforcing the importance of a cooperative setting characterized by a positive, mutually supportive group climate.

SUMMARY

Reinforcement is a needed condition for learning and a powerful procedure used in teaching. The effects of positive reinforcement have been amply documented in the educational literature. In order to foster positive attitudes and behaviors in students, instructors should become sensitive to the ways in which they provide feedback to their students. Praising the desired behavior helps to ensure that it will be repeated.

2

Explaining Through Examples and Models

Explaining is an essential part of teaching. To explain is to make something that is not known or understood by students understandable. Some teachers explain aptly. They seem to get to the heart of the matter with just the right terminology, examples, and organization of ideas. Others, unfortunately, get themselves and others all mixed up. They use terms beyond the level of comprehension of their students; they draw inept or inaccurate analogies, or they employ concepts and principles that cannot be understood by students without their understanding the very thing being explained. Teachers can either go beyond students' comprehension, or they can bore their students by giving ideas beneath the level of student expectations.

An educational system is basically a communication system. It involves a flow of information from the *transmitter* (teacher) to the *receiver* (student) by going through *channels* (language). The transmitter and receiver must agree on the definitions used in the communication process in order to communicate. Therefore, no matter how scholarly the teacher's explanations may be, they are to no advantage to the student if they do not communicate meaning, clarify an issue, or help to relate to previous experiences.

USE OF EXAMPLES

The most common way that teachers explain is by the use of examples. Examples are necessary to clarify, verify, or substantiate concepts. An example helps the student to understand the nature or character of the issue being examined. It may be a smaller part of the issue. An example is, in fact, a sample of the whole. Suppose we wanted to explain to students that all body actions are dependent on the integrity of the moveable body parts. One example, or part of this generalization, would be that hip and knee joints must be altered from flexion to extension in order for a person to stand erect. The effective use of examples includes the following suggestions.

Begin with Simple Examples and Progress to More Complex Ones

By simple we mean what is simple to the student, not to the teacher. There are times when an extreme example may better illustrate a point rather than a more subtle one. To help students to understand and recognize behavior, it may be easier to recognize symptoms in a patient hospitalized specifically because of depression where the symptoms of sleeplessness, anorexia, muteness, and immobility are pronounced rather than expecting the student to recognize the more subtle symptoms of a postpartum depression. Another example might include using, as illustration of principles, simple nursing measures to relieve sleeplessness rather than the more sophisticated measures required for the patient with complex nursing problems.

Select Examples Relevant to Students' Experience and Knowledge

This follows the oft-repeated principle of learning—that of proceeding from the known to the unknown. The use of simple, everyday examples can illustrate scientific principles in easy, understandable terms and assist in comprehension, retention, and transfer of such principles. Suppose we wanted to understand the generalization that protein matter coagulates faster when wet heat is used rather than dry heat. By using an example well known to all students, such as it takes less time to boil an egg than bake one, we are selecting from an experience common to all students. In discussing the family as a sociological unit, if we draw on students' knowledge of families they have known, we are again utilizing their own experiences as examples.

Relate Examples to the Principles or Ideas Being Taught

Informing students that, in most cases, a patient's breathing will be eased if the patient is placed in a sitting position may foster rote learning. If, on the other hand, the principle that breathing is eased when the chest cavity is enlarged by allowing gravity to pull on abdominal organs, as *for example* when a patient is placed in a sitting position, will place the focus on the principle rather than on the example. All teachers have had the experience of having students remember *only* the example while forgetting the principle it illustrated.

Check to See if the Objectives of the Lesson Have Been Achieved by Asking Students to Give Examples That Illustrate the Main Point

This feedback mechanism allows the teacher to ascertain if students understand the main points or principles of a given concept under discussion. Asking students to share experiences that exemplify the concept under consideration not only helps other students to broaden their understanding, but reinforces learnings and promotes transfer.

USE OF EXAMPLES TO GENERALIZE

When students learn to generalize, they are essentially organizing their experiences so that they are meaningful and useful to them. Such organization is important in terms of both retention and transfer. Generalizations can be developed in two ways. The first is by deduction, when a generalization or rule is given to a student and the student deduces examples from the generalization. One such example would be if students were told that an individual whose circulatory system is able to compensate for a decrease in oxygen supply by increasing blood flow is better able to tolerate hypoxia than a patient whose circulatory response is defective or lacking. Following this generalization, students would be asked to *deduce* examples that illustrate this principle.

In the inductive process, the student begins with a set of observations and, based on observations, develops or induces a generalization or principle to predict or explain the pattern of relationships observed. For example, if the teacher wished students to induce the generalization about toleration of hypoxia, students might care for patients who exemplify the principle, such as a patient who has had a sympathectomy, a patient with generalized atherosclerosis, and so forth.

Both deductive and inductive processes promote learning. Deductive learning assists the student in the testing of theory and its application to the solution of problems. Inductive learning helps the student to generalize concepts and theories from experience.

Taba (1967) points out that comparing and contrasting examples are effective teaching strategies following content sampling. Here students are asked to seek similarities and differences among examples to find principles and generalizations to assist in the future use of the concepts under discussion. This way of learning to generalize also assists students in organizing material for themselves.

MODELS

The patient care study can be used as a means of comparing the nursing care needs of a specific patient to the specified possible needs as described in a textbook. Viewed in this way, the care study is an example of a larger body of alternative patterns for nursing care. Selection of content for the nursing curriculum can be derived from the nursing care problems selected as representative of the knowledge required for meeting the nursing care needs of many individuals and families (Harms & McDonald, 1966). In this latter example, the problems have been utilized inductively in order to determine the general content for the nursing course. The specific nursing care problems represented by the problem models are utilized as problem-solving vehicles to assist students in the decision-making process.

A model helps the student to integrate data. One specific type of model is the replica. A replica is a scaled construction that reproduces features of the original. It may be scaled down or be a mock-up of the original. The latter is utilized when something small, for example, a cell, is made more tangible and understandable when blown up. The large replica of the human cell, designed and constructed by a pharmaceutical company, helps the viewer to see relationships of the individual parts, which a microscopic picture or flat plate could never accomplish. Models of this type are frequently used in teaching to assist students in viewing parts of the body not readily seen in perspective without this aid. For example, a mock-up of the human ear is used to illustrate the flow of fluid when the outer canal is irrigated. The replica serves as a pictorial or physical representation of parts or the total under inquiry. The replica serves mainly to describe a static condition, a thing, or a dynamic system at a particular instant of time. The scaled down or scaled upward model can be worked with more easily than the object or system it represents.

Another type of model is termed *analog* model. An analog employs the properties of a familiar system in order to represent the properties of the system under inquiry. It utilizes analogy for explaining something by comparing it with something else. DeWalt and Haines (1969) utilized Selye's stress model to study and explain the effects of stressors on healthy oral mucosa and in predicting the result of specified nursing interventions. The analog model is frequently used in research. The comparison of the human brain to a computer model has been made in order to guide the systematic inquiry of human problem solving (Hovland, 1966). The behavioral sciences have modeled their inquiry by comparison with biological science models. To further clarify, suppose that biological theory of cell growth were used as a model for social growth. Relatively precise meaning has been given to anabolic and catabolic pro cesses in cell growth theory. By giving correspondingly precise meaning to the building and deteriorating processes of human institutions, a one-to-one correspondence is approximated, and we would have the necessary conditions for using cell growth theory as a model for institutional theory. The analog model, unlike the replica, can be utilized effectively to describe, explain, and represent dynamic systems. It is more general than the replica, and as such it can be representative of many different processes.

The third type of model is the symbolic model, which is most frequently utilized in teaching. Symbolic models are intangible except as sounds from a speaker or words on a paper. Words are symbolic models as the word brings the image of what it conveys to the receiver. Mathematical symbols and formulas likewise constitute symbolic models.

USE OF SELF AS ROLE MODEL

In addition to the use of models to explain and clarify teaching, the use of self as a role model in the teaching of nursing cannot be underestimated. Learning from role models is called identification.

Identification has long been prominent in theories of socialization because it explains how individuals learn new behavior and social roles. A number of principles have been proposed for the choice of a model for identification. Secord and Backman (1964) point out that persons may be chosen as models because they frequently reward the learner or because the learner experiences vicarious rewards from their model. The nursing instructor who is praised by a patient or is observed to have assisted in providing comfort to a patient may be selected as a role model by the nursing student who vicariously receives pleasure from the instructor's nursing skill. Persons may be chosen as models because they are envied as recipients of rewards from others. Finally, persons may be chosen as models because the learner perceives traits in the model similar to his or her own.

Mager (1968) points out that modeling behavior is exceedingly important in the achievement of attitude objectives. The often stated phrase "Actions speak louder than words" is relevant here. Paticularly in the clinical area, nursing instructors have the opportunity to behave in ways in which they wish their students to behave. Instructors are truly the living audiovisual examples of what they are trying to convey to their students.

ILLUSTRATIONS

The old cliché "A picture is worth a thousand words" is well known to all. The need for illustration is inherent in the teaching process. Illustrations not only supply missing objects or aspects of a given topic, but they eliminate the need for a continuous effort to recall what has been said before. How would you describe correct body mechanics for lifting an object from the floor by using words alone? Imagine having to give your students a mental picture of the lower intestinal tract without using diagrams or illustrations.

The age of television has emphasized this as a visual age. McLuhan and Fiore (1967) make a strong point that most people find it difficult to understand purely verbal concepts. In general, people feel more secure when things are visible and they can see for themselves. Visual memories are longer than auditory memories.

The use of photographs, videotapes, diagrams, slides, and transparencies all enrich the teaching-learning process. There is much material from which to choose; so much material, in fact, that it can cause the nursing instructor to become confused and perplexed in selecting appropriate materials to illustrate the principles being taught. The National Medical Audiovisual Center is a federal agency that can provide help to nursing faculty. The overall mission of the National Medical

Audiovisual Center is to improve the quality and use of biomedical audiovisual materials in schools for the health professions (Sparks & Mitchell, 1978). The development of prototype instructional materials is encouraged, and products that are deemed to be of high quality are distributed. A listing of audiovisual instructional materials can be obtained from the National Medical Audiovisual Center (Annex), Station K, Atlanta, Georgia 30324.

SUMMARY

Effective teaching requires effective communication. The use of examples, models, and illustrations assists students in proceeding from what they know and have experienced to something new. Examples help students to apply principles and generalizations to specific instances.

3

Using Simulation
and Games

Simulation and games for teaching have been used for many years. War games date back centuries and are still used for training military personnel. Most readers are probably familiar with the use of flight simulators for training military and commercial pilots, space simulators for training astronauts, and automobile simulators for driver education.

The idea of using simulation and games in formal education is also not a new one. Games were mentioned in educational writings as early as 1775 (Knight, 1949). James (1908) encouraged teachers to make learning more activity oriented. More recently, other educators have argued that vicarious experience and acting on what has been learned are important parts of the total learning situation (Carlson, 1969). Common sense support for the value of experiential learning techniques is found in the writings of Mark Twain who said, "A fellow who takes a bull by the tail once gets as much as sixty or seventy times the information as one who doesn't."

Such views require that education shift its focus from the mere transmission of content to one of bringing theory and real-life experiences closer together. Further, with the recognition of a great proliferation of knowledge it becomes important to help learners develop skills of inquiry and problem solving that will increase their effectiveness in coping with future situations. Increasingly, then, experiential techniques, including simulations and games became a part of the educational scene.

The first formal use of simulation games in education was in 1959

(Rossi & Briddle, 1966). By 1964, the majority of graduate schools of business had made management games a part of their standard curricula (Dale & Klassen, 1964). Simulation techniques have been used in education of medical students since the mid-1960s (Barrows, 1968; Hoban, 1978). Nursing educators have also used simulation techniques for many years, although the term, simulation, was not used until recently. Examples include the practice of basic skills in such simulated settings as skills laboratories, use of simulated nursing stations in a laboratory setting, and the use of role playing to gain insight into the feelings of others and for learning and practicing interpersonal, problem-solving, and crisis intervention skills. More recently, there have been a number of textbooks and articles written by nursing educators that specifically discuss the use of simulation and games. Many of them will be cited throughout this chapter.

This chapter focuses on the application of simulation and games to nursing education. Terms are defined early to distinguish between the two. Simulation and games are then discussed together in the area of potential educational benefits since previous writings often have not made a clear distinction between the two. After this initial common discussion, simulation and games are covered separately. Examples are given, processes identified, and uses established. The chapter ends with a listing of limitations and concerns applicable to both simulation and games.

DEFINITIONS

It is apparent when reading about simulations and games that there is much inconsistency about the use of the two terms. Often the terms are used together, that is, simulation games or simulation/games, although what is being discussed is clearly one or the other but not both, or both are discussed without identifying which is which. Robinson (1966) uses the terms interchangeably. Coleman (1970) defines the terms differently. Other authors provide guidance in developing definitions that help to clarify and distinguish between the two terms (Carlson, 1969; Tansey & Unwin, 1969; Raser, 1969; Abt, 1971; Curtis & Rothert, 1972; Cruickshank, 1977; Rockler, 1978; McKeachie, 1978; Thiagarajan & Stolovich, 1978; Cooper, 1979). Following is a synthesis from these resources of the two terms as they will be used in this chapter in relation to educational application.

SIMULATION: A realistic representation (model) of the structure or dynamics of a real thing or process with which the participant, as an active part of the experience, interacts with persons or things in the environment, applies previously learned knowledge to make responses (decisions and actions) to deal with a problem or situation, and receives feedback about responses without the direct real-life consequences.

GAME: An activity governed by precise rules that involves varying degrees of chance or risk and one or more players who compete (with self, the game, one another, or a computer) through the use of knowledge, skill, strength, or luck in an attempt to reach a specified goal (gain an intrinsic or extrinsic reward).

SIMULATION GAME: An activity that incorporates the characteristics of *both* a simulation and a game; a game that also models some real-life situation or process.

It is apparent, then, that all games are not simulations; all simulations are not games; and an experience may be both a simulation and a game depending on its specific characteristics. With simulation there is a distinct and explicit analogy between the activity and real life, while in gaming, which is not also a simulation, that analogy with real life may be a distant abstraction. Many games bear little or no resemblance to actual life processes and situations even though they may use social interaction as a mechanism of play as well as active participation of the student. In this chapter, when the term simulation is used, it will include both nongame simulations and simulation games; when the term game is used it will be referring to nonsimulation games only.

It may be helpful to view learning experiences on a continuum such as that depicted by Table 3-1. It reflects levels of learning from the two extremes—concrete and abstract—and is a combination and adaptation of the ideas presented previously by Dale (1969) and Russell (1974).

Nonsimulation games may fit at different levels of this continuum, depending on the unique characteristics of each game, but all are closer to more abstract experiences. Many games are highly abstract, using auditory or visual stimuli only (e.g., word games, spelling games, question-and-answer games, crossword puzzles, and card games). Others are more concrete as they move closer to representing real-life processes and activities, for example, computer or group problem-solving games. Those activities that can be classified as simulations and simulation games fall closer to the level of concrete experiences. However, direct involvement in a contrived experience can itself represent varying degrees of closeness to reality. For example, practicing a skill, such as preparing and starting an intravenous infusion, could be accomplished at varying degrees of simulation. One level is practice without the use of

Table 3-1
Levels of Experience

Concrete Experiences

1. Direct participation in real-life events (clinical experience)

2. Direct involvement in a contrived experience in an environment that is a representation of reality (simulation: role playing, practice of skills, some games)

3. Direct observation of an actual experience or demonstration (field trips, demonstrations, observer of dramatizations or clinical practice)

4. Indirect perception of experiences by visual representation (filmstrips, movies, videotape, television, exhibits, photographs)

5. Indirect perception of experiences by audiorepresentation (records, audiotapes, sound tracks)

6. Reading descriptions of experiences (printed matter: texts, articles, case studies)

7. Hearing descriptions of experiences (lectures, audiotape, discussion)

Abstract Experiences

SOURCE: Adapted from Russell, J. D. Figure E, *Modular instruction*. Minneapolis, Burgess Publishing Co., 1974. Used by permission.

a mannikin; another is practice using a mannikin without simulated veins; another is practice on a simulator with veins; and the next would be practice on a simulated patient (a peer or someone else trained to behave and respond like a patient). Each has certain values in relation to learning and level of anxiety experienced by the student. For example, a beginning student may gain more, initially, by working with a mannikin rather than a simulated patient since level of stress is likely to be increased when practicing on a real person.

POTENTIAL EDUCATIONAL BENEFITS OF USING SIMULATION AND GAMING

Many authors have described the benefits associated with using simulation or games, or both. Those from Greenblat (cited in Wolf & Duffy, 1979) are summarized below:

1. Motivation and interest in the topic, course, and learning in general are increased due to direct involvement and active participation of the student.

2. Cognitive learning, including factual information, concepts, principles, and decision-making skills, is improved.

3. Later course work is more meaningful, since students are led to more sophisticated and relevant inquiry during those experiences following the use of simulation/gaming.
4. Affective learning associated with the subject matter is improved by altering students' attitudes and perceptions of issues and people and increasing their empathy and insight into others different from themselves.
5. General affective learning is improved by increasing each student's self-awareness and sense of personal effectiveness.
6. Classroom structure and interactional patterns are improved by promoting good student–teacher relations, encouraging the free exploration of ideas, decreasing the punitive role of the teacher, increasing student autonomy in the learning situation, and increasing exchange of ideas among different types of students.

There is wide support for the use of simulation and gaming if the aims are to motivate students, change attitudes, and alter interactional patterns. Gordan (1970, p. 200) states that there is now general agreement that "simulation/gaming has its greatest measurable effect in the area of attitudes." He goes on to say, however, that most of the research in this area has occurred at the primary and secondary school levels. McKeachie (1978) agrees that research is sparse in higher education settings.

A few nursing studies are available that provide data about affective gains from the use of simulation and gaming in higher education. They are summarized below:

1. Shaffer and Pfeiffer (1978) concluded that students using videotaped simulations of critical incidents were more involved and participated at a significantly higher level than the students using written materials only.
2. Stuck and Manatt (1970) reported higher levels of motivation in a group using simulation techniques.
3. In their use of the simulation game, "Mental Hospital," Laszlo and McKenzie (1979) found that the personnel who participated changed their attitudes toward patients in mental hospitals in the direction of greater sensitivity and that they were more highly motivated to obtain further information about patient rights.
4. Godejohn, Taylor, Muhlenkamp, and Blaesser (1975) found that the use of two simulation games produced significant decreases in authoritarianism and social restrictiveness scores on a scale measuring opinions about mental illness, while the scores for the control group

remained the same. They concluded that this data provided compelling evidence to support the use of simulation games for changing attitudes toward mental illness.

In contrast to the area of affective gains from the use of simulation and gaming, there is less agreement about the benefits to cognitive learning. Before the 1960s, increased interest and involvement of students using simulation and games were frequently considered to be adequate evidence that learning had occurred (Boocock & Schild, 1968). However, the reports during that period were primarily descriptive in nature, including little statistical validation of learning effects. It is generally agreed that there is a lack of evidence to support the claims for improved cognitive learning (Cherryholmes, 1966; Glazier, 1970). Reiser (1981) believes that this is due to a lack of systematic development of simulation games, the failure to use them as an integral part of an instructional program, and the absence of research about the unique attributes of simulation games which would increase their effectiveness.

Typically, the research that has been done compares simulation and games with traditional classroom instruction techniques. Some of the results indicate that there is no difference in the amount of learning between the two (McKeachie, 1978; Lewis, et al., 1974; Reiser, 1981; Shaffer & Pfeiffer, 1978). For example, Shaffer and Pfeiffer concluded that there was no significant difference in cognitive learning between the use of traditional methods and the use of videotaped simulations in preparing baccalaureate nursing students for home visits. At the same time, it is important to note that such results also indicate that the use of this alternative approach was no less effective than the traditional methods.

There are several studies available in different areas that indicate the superiority of simulation and gaming techniques over traditional methods. For example, Baker (1968) found that learning in history was improved with a pre–Civil War simulation; Wing (1968) reported that with a computerized game there was considerably less time investment required to achieve the same amount of learning; and Farran (1968) found that the performance of underachievers was improved in the areas of learning content, strategic decision making, relational thinking, and planning. In medical education, Penta and Kofman (1973) reported that an experimental group, using eye and heart sound simulators for developing skills of physical diagnosis, scored significantly higher on an objective test than the group not using the simulators.

Examples of studies in nursing education that show simulation techniques to be superior to traditional methods for cognitive learning are as follows:

1. Stuck and Manatt (1970) determined that both an economy of time and improved cognitive learning occurred in a group using audiotutorial simulation.
2. McIntyre, McDonald, Bailey, and Claus (1972) found that a group using written simulations had significantly higher scores on the criterion measures of communication and data-gathering skills and the selection of beneficial items.
3. Laszlo and McKenzie (1979) found that participants who gained "experience" as mental hospital patients through a simulation game gained significant increase in knowledge about patient rights.
4. Jeffers and Christensen (1979) demonstrated the value of simulation in the development of clinical observational skills and a smoother transition into an actual leadership experience.

Research findings about the effectiveness of computer simulations are given in Chapter 14.

Research into the advantages and limitations of simulations and games as educational tools is ongoing. The emphasis is on identifying techniques that will test the effectiveness and impact of these strategies (Belch, 1973). In his review of studies evaluating the effectiveness of simulations and games, Cherryholmes (1966) contends that simulation produces effects that have not yet been specified or measured. It is widely accepted that simulation games work but the precise knowledge about how and why they work is needed (Boocock & Schild, 1968).

SIMULATION

Several factors call for the use of alternative strategies in nursing education, particularly for the clinical component. Critics of nursing education at the college and university levels contend that it is too theoretically based, that students have inadequate clinical experience, and that much of what is taught is inconsistent with the "real" world of nursing. Issues associated with teaching in the clinical area include (1) the need for close supervision especially at the early skill development stage, thus making it more costly and time-consuming; (2) the decreasing availability of clinical facilities for student experience due to an increase in the numbers and varieties of students in the health professions; (3) the unpredictability of clinical experiences, thus an inability at times to plan specific experiences desired for all students; (4) the concern for client safety and comfort; and (5) the difficulty with precise evaluation of performance in the clinical setting.

These factors can be at least partially dealt with through the use of simulation as a strategy for teaching and evaluation. In addition, simulation techniques can be used in an attempt to incorporate known principles of learning (Cross, 1976) related to motivation, active participation, relevance and transfer of learning, individual discovery of knowledge, and feedback about performance.

Further justification for the use of experiential techniques with nursing students is found in the recognition that most students in nursing programs are of the "sensing-feeling" type (Bradshaw, 1978, p. 33). Bradshaw states:

> One of the major characteristics of this group appears to be their affinity for learning through the use of their senses. These persons are more comfortable and able to perceive their world more clearly through their sense of touch, feel, smell, sight, and taste. They are often categorized as 'concrete' thinkers because they determine the reality of a thing by whether it can be taken in through the senses. 'Experiencing' becomes the key word and a major activity through which an instructor can reach many students without resorting to telling.

Types of Simulation

In their writings on the use of simulations in the health professions, Maatsch and Gordan (1978) identified five types of simulation. Their classification has been somewhat modified and expanded for use in this chapter and includes (1) written simulations, (2) role played simulations, (3) audiovisually mediated simulations, (4) physical simulators, (5) live simulated patients, (6) computer simulations, and (7) gamed simulations. These simulation types are not mutually exclusive. One or more may be incorporated into any single activity. However, each will be discussed separately for the sake of simplicity.

Written Simulation.   A written simulation is a paper-and-pencil presentation of actual problems or cases about which the student must make decisions as if performing in the situation. With each decision the student receives feedback about the effects of that action and incorporates that information into the next decision. The progression of events follows that established by the actual situation. Written simulation includes "in-basket" techniques and the clinical problem-solving technique, patient management problem (PMP).

The in-basket technique.   This written simulation technique requires the participant to take action on various letters, papers, and memos as if they were arriving in the incoming mail (Sylvester, 1974). Participants decide what they would do, share their decisions and the rationale for them with others, and receive feedback about the anticipated effects of each decision. Such activities are particularly useful when teaching and evaluating the application of principles of management.

"You are Barbara Jordan" is an example of an in-basket exercise that can be used to teach or evaluate decision making in nursing service administration (Cooper, 1979). The items appearing in the in-basket are typical of those that need the attention of any nursing service administrator, ranging from routine scheduling problems to emergency situations. Areas of particular emphasis include the need to establish priorities, ability to delegate responsibility, and analysis of factors that affect decision making in an administrative capacity.

The patient management problem.   A PMP is a paper-and-pencil branched programmed activity simulating the decision-making process as if in an actual patient encounter.

It was originally developed for use in medical education and licensure (Hubbard, et al., 1965; McGuire & Babbott, 1967) and was first introduced to nursing education by de Tornyay (1968) with the "simulated clinical nursing problem test." The PMP can be used either for teaching or evaluating problem-solving skills, including making judgments in the clinical area. de Tornyay (1968) believes that they are especially helpful for emphasizing problem-solving skills that cannot be adequately measured by traditional multiple-choice test items and for providing predictions about a student's future clinical performance.

McGuire and Babbott (1967) outline five essential characteristics of a clinical problem which claims to simulate a real patient encounter:

1. The problem must be presented in a realistic manner with the amount and type of information that would be available to the student on the encounter with the client.
2. It must require a series of sequential, interdependent decisions on the part of the participant as would be reflected in the actual resolution of a problem.
3. Each decision must be followed by the receipt of realistic information about the results of the decision, which can then be used in making subsequent decisions.
4. The format must be such that an ineffective or harmful decision cannot be retracted after the results of a decision are known.

5. It must allow for different approaches for dealing with the problem and variable patient responses in relation to each approach.

The key process, then, is receipt of baseline information, decision, feedback about decision (more information), subsequent decision, and so forth. Students have an opportunity to select from among relevant and irrelevant and beneficial and harmful options. Thus, each student can follow a different path to obtain additional information and solve the problem. The mechanism also provides for remediation or termination of the activity (depending on whether the PMP is being used for teaching or for evaluation) should the student select an alternative that is inappropriate or dangerous.

Nursing literature contains several descriptions of the use of the PMP at various levels of nursing education. Curtis and Rothert (1972) describe the use of a written simulation with sophomore nursing students for focusing on the use of various data sources in assessing a client. They also used 8-mm films, slides, and hospital records as adjuncts to the written program to provide a more realistic visual representation of patient and surroundings. The authors report a high degree of cognitive involvement of the participants, the value of the media for motivating the students, and the value of the written simulation as a tool for self-assessment.

Research by McIntyre and associates (1972) regarding the effectiveness of written simulations has been cited previously. In a related article, Page and Saunders (1978) describe their experience with a written simulation for teaching and evaluating the use of the assessment and planning phases of the nursing process to first year nursing students. They conclude that the written simulation has value as a teaching/learning tool by complementing existing methods and dealing with constraints associated with teaching in the actual clinical setting, for example, distractions and client safety.

Although definitive conclusions cannot be drawn regarding the effectiveness of the PMP, two studies in nurse practitioner programs (Sherman et al., 1979; Holzemer et al., 1981) support the PMP as a tool for the measurement of clinical problem solving/decision making. Continuing efforts are expected to be made toward perfecting the design of PMPs with further testing of their reliability and validity.

Three other reports in the nursing literature are worthy of note at this time. Although they do not report on the use of the PMP as described above, the procedures are somewhat related and reflect an effort to facilitate the development of problem-solving skills. All also appear to be closely related to the well-known case study method. O'Connell and Bates (1976) describe the use of the case history to promote students' abilities to select, analyze, interpret, and utilize information in an active, practice-oriented way. Wales and Hageman (1979) report on the use of "Guided Design Systems" with teams of graduate students for teaching systematic decision-making skills using both knowledge and values. After decisions are made and feedback is received, the students are informed about what actually happened in the real situation. The retrospective examination of an actual problem was also used by Erickson and Borgmeyer (1979) with graduate students in nursing service administration. Through the use of a systems model, they analyze the manner in which a situation has been handled by looking at alternative solutions and options and considering value, feasibility, and patient safety and satisfaction.

Role Played Simulation.   Role playing is a simulation technique in which one person assumes the role of another. Therefore, participants who are involved in simulations that call upon them to respond as themselves (such as with PMPs just discussed) are not involved in role playing. It should be pointed out, however, that role played simulations have less fidelity with reality than those in which participants deal with problems as themselves.

A few major points, only, will be made about the use of role playing. For the reader who desires more detail about either the development or use of role playing situations, Schweer (1972) and Shaftel and Shaftel (1967) may be useful.

The primary purpose of role playing is to help participants and observers gain new perceptions about human relationships—particularly insights and empathy into the behaviors and feelings of people who are different from themselves. Only willing players should be selected, since they must be able to become involved in the role without being threatened or exposed by it. The technique forces the participant to think about the person whose role is assumed. It has been used for many years in psychiatric nursing and is often a part of various exercises attempting to provide an essence of reality.

Role played simulation may be partly structured or completely spontaneous once roles have been assigned. Typically, it involves the use of a critical incident or problem situation depicting conflict between persons, such as with a nurse and a noncompliant client, in which participants play specific roles in the way that they visualize each person would react. Usually, a limited number of the members in a group are involved in the role play while the remaining members act as observers. Specific tasks may be assigned to observers in order to focus their attention on desired aspects of the situation.

The length of the role play itself varies but typically lasts from 5 to 15 minutes. Upon termination of the role play, the participants and observers analyze what occurred, what feelings were generated, what insights were gained, why things happened as they did, and how the situation is related to reality. The procedure usually includes asking particpants to discuss their feelings about the roles and observations about interactions before asking observers to enter into the discussion. It is important to focus criticisms on the role played and the problem presented rather than on the person playing the role. Analysis and discussion may be aided by being able to replay the role played situation; therefore, videotaping could be used if more precise recall of the incident is desired.

An example of a role played simulation used with undergraduate students is provided by Daniel, Eigsti, and McGuire (1977). In their desire to minimize reality shock in case load management in community health, they used a 3-hour simulated exercise preceded by other assignments designed to familiarize the students with roles of various categories of community health personnel. The students, groups of six in assigned roles of supervisor, team leader, public health nurse with a baccalaureate degree, registered nurse without a degree, licensed practical nurse, and home health aide, must deal with a task involving caseload management. Once the group has completed the task, each group presents its plan and rationale to another group. The authors feel that it has been helpful for presenting a total picture of a community health agency and presenting a more realistic picture of caseload management.

Another example is one used at the graduate level (Keller & MacCormick, 1980). Graduate students who are learning about curriculum development are placed in faculty roles by random drawing and make up a task group with the responsibility for developing a masters and a doctoral program in nursing. The simulation lasts for the entire semester and culminates with a report about the programs that have been developed to the real faculty in the setting.

Audiovisually Mediated Simulation.   A simulation in this category uses audiovisual media to present a problem, case, or task; to represent some aspect of an interpersonal encounter; or to provide an avenue for analysis of a role played or other simulated situation. Such mediated situations may be used either for teaching or evaluation.

Videotaped simulation.   An often used audiovisually mediated simulation is that using videotape. Two types are common: those representing interpersonal relations and interviewing skills and those used in teacher training. Those used in the area of interpersonal relations and interviewing skills frequently make use of an interview or problem situation that is acted by a trained "patient" or professional in the area being exhibited. The patient presents verbal and nonverbal cues to which the students are asked to state or demonstrate what their verbal and nonverbal responses would be. Students may be either asked to give free responses to each situation or required to select from a list of alternatives. When the student is forced to select from a given list of alternatives, patient responses to each can be prepared for continued dramatization of the interview situation so that the student receives immediate feedback about effects of actions.

Videotaped simulation of this type is often used for evaluation and testing. Rogers (1976) used videotaped sequences focusing on a particular behavior to validate registered nurse competence in interpersonal skills. The student is asked to write verbal and nonverbal responses to each behavior and to give the rationale for responses. Responses are evaluated as most therapeutic, appropriate, and least therapeutic with competence determined by 75 percent or more of student responses in the first two categories.

In another testing situation Richards, Jones, Nichols, Richardson, Riley, and Swinson (1981) developed videocassette testing programs of situations frequently encountered in an acute care psychiatric setting. There is a dramatization of four interview situations to which the student is asked to respond, write a description of the observed behavior for charting, identify major patient problems and appropriate actions, write a diagnostic label of the behavior, and list common treatment modalities. Criteria are used to evaluate the student's responses to each episode and the results used as 50 percent of the clinical grade. The authors believe that the results provide a more accurate indicator of ability than do traditional methods of evaluating clinical performance.

Variations of the interview situation described above are used by Rynerson (1980) and Eggert (1975) for teaching and evaluation. Rynerson describes the use of videotaped peer interviews with senior students in a psychosocial nursing course. Upon completion, the videotapes are reviewed by the instructor with the two students to discuss their thoughts, feelings, images, sensations, and so forth. The instructor is nonjudgmental and follows the review with a discussion of how to work through thoughts and feelings aroused by the experience. The author reports that the anxiety level of most students has been decreased by this experience.

Eggert (1975) describes the use of a videotaped interview between peers for challenge exams in interpersonal skills. The "patient" is expected to discuss a real problem for which the student provides counseling. A rating guide is then used to determine level of performance.

Other examples of videotaped simulation are the videotaping of a dressing change on a "patient" for later evaluation by self, peers, and teacher (Memmer, 1979); illustrations of home health care (Steiner & Rothenberg, 1980); and critical incidents in typical home visits for teaching nursing process related to the home visit (Shaffer & Pfeiffer, 1980). In each situation, the videotape can be interrupted at any point for discussion.

The teacher training technique, microteaching, is another variation of videotaped simulation. Microteaching technique was originated by Allen and Ryan (1969) and adapted to the preparation of nursing instructors by de Tornyay and Searight (1968). In microteaching the student teacher presents small segments of a lesson to a few students during a short time period for the purpose of practicing a single component of teaching, such as questioning (McKeachie, 1978). With the focus on process rather than content, the sessions provide a controlled setting in which skills can be practiced without the complexities and responsibilities associated with the classroom or clinical setting. Review of the videotape with feedback about teaching behaviors from peers and instructor provide the teacher trainee with the opportunity to gain a better perspective of self by evaluating teaching methods, mannerisms, speech patterns, and other skills and behaviors relative to teaching (Zides, 1974). Other advantages include increased flexibility and economy of time, effort, and money (de Tornyay & Searight, 1968).

In other adaptations of the technique, microteaching has been used to teach an extension course in distant locations from the main campus (Davis & Eaton, 1974) and as part of an elective course in which students are preparing to teach a group of patients (Chapman, 1978). In these two applications, student responses are reported to be highly positive with the associated values of decreased level of anxiety, increased level of confidence, and increased attention by students to specific behaviors important to teaching a group.

Electronic reproductions.   This category of audiovisually mediated simulation includes the audio reproductions of human cardiac and respiratory sounds. Such reproductions can be used to teach and evaluate students who are learning basic and advanced physical assessment skills and to use tools for monitoring various body processes, such as fetal heart tones during pregnancy and labor. One technique for adding realism is to have the student place the stethoscope directly on the playback unit to focus attention, increase concentration ability, and remove distractions.

Physical Simulators.   This category includes the use of three-dimensional lifelike models of part or all of the human body to teach or evaluate specific clinical skills. They provide the student with a means of learning, practicing, and repracticing. The goal is to increase student confidence and competence in the performance of clinical skills for later application to the clinical setting. Another advantage is the increased patient safety and comfort when students are more proficient. When used for evaluation, the student can be either observed directly or the performance videotaped for later viewing by the teacher.

A wide variety of models of the human body is currently available, including some designed to aid in the development of specific skills, such as enema administration, urinary catheterization, breast examination, administration of injections, and colostomy care. Their approximation to reality varies from simple models to be practiced on to those that provide some type of response to student actions. The well-known "Mrs. Chase" is an example of the former, allowing students to practice such procedures as bed baths and positioning. A more sophisticated model is the intravenous (IV) injection arm, which is used to do venipunctures, give IV injections, and administer IV fluids. It provides a more realistic experience as there is a "blood" return and an opportunity to actually inject fluids into the simulated veins. Even more sophisticated computerized robots have been used for some time in the education of medical students (Denson & Abrahamson, 1969; Barrows & Abrahamson, 1964). Sim-One, a computerized robot developed by the medical school at the University of Southern California, is used to train residents in anesthesia administration. It simulates human reaction—changes in color, respirations, blood pressure, heart action—in response to the administration of drugs and gases, thus providing a risk free mechanism for the practice of complex skills. Another robot, Harvey, is an animated mannikin that can simulate cardiovascular disease states (Hoban, 1978). Harvey can be programmed to exhibit eye grounds, pupillary reactions, aging, stroke, and alterations in blood pressure. Such simulators, besides providing the risk-free setting, also furnish immediate feedback to the student, allow a student to progress at his or her own rate, and permit individual acts to be repeated as often as necessary.

There are numerous reports in the nursing literature about the settings in which less sophisticated physical simulators are used. Representative of these are the Clinical Simulation Laboratory at the University of Texas (Allen, 1974); the Skills Laboratory at San Jose State University (Rochin & Thompson, 1975); the self-instructional laboratory at the University of Wisconsin (Hoose, 1976); and the practice laboratory at the University of Connecticut (Infante, 1981). There have been no reports in the nursing literature about the use of robots like Sim-One and Harvey, perhaps because of the high costs of these innovations. Should funding be obtainable, such robots offer the same advantages to nursing education, especially in the area of nurse practitioner training, as they do for medical education.

Live Simulated Patients. This type of simulation, useful for either teaching or evaluating, involves the use of persons trained to act in the role of the patient (Hoban, 1978). It is a technique that has been used for some time in medical education (Barrows, 1968, 1971). The person playing the role of the patient is directed to exhibit certain clinical behaviors, provide a specific history, respond in certain interpersonal ways during an encounter with a student, or give students feedback about performance of skills. The episode is also sometimes videotaped or attended by an objective observer for the purpose of providing feedback about student behaviors.

The "patient" may be played by a peer, drama student, paid actor, or faculty member. For example, Zides (1974) reports that faculty members were used to demonstrate certain clinical symptoms for student observation. Others (Beyers et al., 1972; Rochin & Thompson, 1975) describe the use of peers acting as the patient for the practice of psychomotor skills. Peers also serve as patients during a 2-day workshop that simulates a hospital day and is intended to improve the transition from the practice lab to the actual setting (Sullivan et al., 1977). Actors have been used to prepare videotapes for simulated nursing rounds intended to sharpen observational skills (Jeffers & Christensen, 1979) and to provide students with practice in interviewing and learning about heart and respiratory sounds (Lincoln et al., 1978). The sequence of events identified in the latter situation was observation of a videotape demonstrating assessment, lecture-discussion, supervised practice with a peer, practice with a simulated patient, and assessment of real patients. The result of decreased fear of making mistakes or harming the patient supports the use of this technique for initial skill development.

Computer Simulation. Simulations of this type use a computer to present cases, provide information requested by the student, incorporate decisions made, and provide feedback to the student about the effects of decisions. Both psychomotor and cognitive decisions can be incorporated into computer simulations. For example, the computerized robots discussed in the section on physical simulators are programmed to respond in certain ways to specific student actions. However, most computer simulations in medical and nursing education involve the simulation of patient care problems similar to the patient management problems discussed in the section on written simulations. Typically, the computer presents a patient situation to the student who requests additional information, makes responses, intervenes, and receives feedback about the consequences of decisions made. Thus, the student gains practice in clinical decision making and judgment without the fear of doing something wrong or harming a patient. (See Chapter 14 for further discussion of computer simulation.)

Gamed Simulation.   This category of simulation includes those activities that have the characteristics of both a game and a simulation, as defined at the beginning of this chapter. Thus, a gamed simulation (or a simulation game) must be active and interactive in a problem situation, operated according to set rules, and involve an element of competition in reaching the specified goal. It can involve winners and losers; however, the gamed simulation can be designed so that everyone who is involved in the activity wins if the specified goal is achieved. Simulation activities that require game boards, dice, cards, and so forth are also referred to as simulation games, although they may not have other gamelike characteristics.

Research by Laszlo and McKenzie (1979) and Godejohn, Taylor, Muhlenkamp, and Blaesser (1975) about their use of simulation games has been cited previously (see pages 27 and 29). A brief description of the simulation games used by Laszlo and McKenzie and others is presented in summary form (Table 3-2) as examples of what is available. A complete example of one simulation game is given in Appendix 1. Other simulation games that are commercially available can be located in guides (Horn & Zuckerman, 1977; Belch, 1973), catalogs (Sim-Ed, 1978), or individual publications (Wolf & Duffy, 1979).

USING SIMULATION FOR INSTRUCTION

Teaching is primarily concerned with providing information and facilitating concept formation, acquisition of skills, attitudinal change, and problem solving. Hoban and Casberque state, "As a method of clinical instruction, simulations can be used to facilitate (1) learning and retention, (2) transfer of training, (3) understanding, (4) attitude formation, and (5) motivation" (Hoban and Casberque, 1978, pp. 147–148). Simulations provide the student with direct, active experiences, which decrease the need for clinical facilities at the unskilled practice level and increase the student's readiness for application of knowledge and skills to the actual situation. The quality of learning is improved when the student has had previous experience with a situation before confronting

Table 3-2
Examples of Gamed Simulations Suitable for Nursing Education

Title of Gamed Simulation	Availability	Number of Players	Playing Time	Objectives and Description of Activity
Bafá bafá	Simile II P.O. Box 910 Del Mar, CA 92014	12–80	1½ h plus 30 min to discuss	Participants live and cope in a "foreign" culture and are both perpetrators and victims of stereotyping. Demonstrates the phenomenon of culture shock, negative effects of stereotyping, and the development of understanding of reasons behind behaviors.
Synoptics	See Dearth and McKenzie (1975) for complete description	12	40 min play plus 15 min for decision	Deals with role bias and selective perception and the importance of being aware of the perspectives of others. Designed to help health professionals view the delivery of health care from various perspectives. Uses roles of nurse, doctor, and administrator. Observers act as the jury for decisions.
Mental hospital	See Laszlo and McKenzie (1979) for complete description	Varies	Varies	Health personnel participants play the roles of patients in a mental hospital and attempt to earn their discharge and get a job. The goal is to change the attitudes of hospital employees toward increased sensitivity and to increase knowledge about patient rights.
Here comes the judge	See Appendix 1 for complete description, rules, and procedures	3 groups of 3–5 plus observers	Varies	The purpose is to provide group participation for solving nursing problems. Employs the team concept and intergroup cooperation to beat the other team. Designed to take groups through all phases of problem solving and utilize strengths of all members.
Assignment	John Wiley & Sons 605 Third Avenue New York, NY 10158	2–6	40 min to 2 h	Part of LEGS program. The goal is to complete the patient assignment in the least number of moves and to defend each action. Student nurses are given the opportunity to see how advanced planning can conserve energy and provide better patient care (Belch, 1973; Wolf & Duffy, 1979).

it in the work environment. Furthermore, the use of simulations provides desired experiences to all students without having to depend on their availability in the clinical arena.

Simulations deal with systems and processes and the development of complex skills associated with them. Thus, they prepare individuals to make decisions and judge decisions made by others. Simulation is particularly useful when the components of a task are complex and difficult to analyze. It provides the essence of those real-life situations about which strategies must be learned. Ideas are developed and tested in a safe environment without fear of doing something wrong or harming a client. Creative behavior and divergent thinking are encouraged rather than having one "right" answer projected. Decisions and their consequences are studied. The intent is to increase the student's awareness of what the real-life situation will be like and increase the chance for successful performance when the student is in the actual situation. In addition, students may increase their personal sense of competence and confidence in dealing with new situations; gain an awareness that there are many ways to deal with a problem; achieve insight into the behaviors of self and others; increase their tolerance for different points of view; and increase their skill for working with others to solve a problem.

Hoban and Casberque (1978, p. 148) identify four properties that simulations should have in order to be of instructional value. They are:

1. The student should respond sensitively to the stimulus in the simulation. . . .
2. The spatial, tactile, chromatic, mobile, auditory, and/or temporal relationships found in the simulation should be analogous to real life. . . .
3. The fidelity of the critical properties and actual sequence of the activities in the simulation should be sufficient enough to assure that the activity being practiced transfers to real situations. . . .
4. Feedback to the students should provide them with information about the consequences of their actions. . . .

Although each of these properties may be variable in different simulations, all should be present to some degree in every simulation activity. The first property requires that students actively participate in the activity. Simulation is an experiential strategy since it involves a high degree of involvement between the participant and elements in the environment. These elements can be other people, computerized or noncomputerized mannikins, equipment, or a computer program. The participation may be through hands-on involvement (as in the use of models for practice of pelvic or breast examination and colostomy care) or through intellectual involvement (as in the use of written or computerized patient problems to practice decision-making skills). Either way the student is not the passive participant in learning that is sometimes the case with traditional methods.

The second and third properties deal with proximity to reality in relation to physical characteristics, critical elements, and sequence of events. The models used should be as realistic as possible. For example, those models most closely approximating reality, such as computerized robots, provide experiences that give the student a sense of involvement in the actual situation and increase the ability to transfer learning to the real setting. Traditional classroom techniques often deal with what *might* be; on the other hand, simulations such as written and computerized patient problem situations deal with what *is* since students are required to respond as if they were in the real situation.

The fourth property deals with feedback to the student about behaviors during the simulation. Primarily, this involves the student becoming aware of the consequences of actions taken. Hoban and Casberque (1978, p. 148) identify three types of feedback: sensory, direct instructional intervention, and critique. With sensory feedback the students use their own senses to determine the appropriateness of their actions. For example, breast examination models simulate various types of nodules. By examining the breasts, the students receive sensory feedback by locating the nodules and differentiating among the types. With direct feedback, the student is given information about appropriateness of actions taken via a written or mediated instructional package, the instructor, or a person who is playing the role of a patient. For example, the student in a simulated interview situation can receive feedback about verbal or nonverbal behaviors, or the student using a computerized or written patient problem can receive feedback about each action taken. In critique the feedback is given at the end of the simulation. In this way, the student can compare what has been done with what experts in the field or other objective observers would recommend.

The Process of Using Simulation for Instruction

As stated in the definition given previously, an activity is a simulation when it is a realistic representation of an actual situation. It must incorporate the roles, events, and consequences of a real situation or process. It allows a "slice of life" to be discussed, managed, manipulated, and repeated within a condensed time frame for the learning benefits of the participants.

Preliminaries. Simulation activities are best incorporated as one strategy among several as an integral part of an instructional program. Simulation should not be used simply for the sake of using a different approach. As with any other strategy, simulation exercises must be selected and developed because they are expected to provide the most useful mechanism for reaching specific objectives.

Once it is decided that simulation is best to use for certain objectives, the teacher has several tasks to complete. The first, of course, is either to select a simulation activity that is already available or to design one for the purposes desired. A discussion of design is beyond the scope of this chapter; however, other resources are available that provide guidelines. Bevis (1978) provides guidelines for building games; however, the process identified applies to simulations as well. In Horn & Zuckerman (1977) there is a special chapter on design. Other helpful references include Glazier (1970), Stonewater (1978), Thiagarajan & Stolovich (1978), Thiagarajan (1980), and Hoban and Casberque (1978).

Simulations that are commercially available can be located by referring to guides and catalogs already mentioned (see page 39). Simulations in a variety of subject areas, including health and medicine, are available. Although those specifically designed for nursing are limited, some that are designed for other related areas may be useful for specific objectives that are common to several health care fields.

Any educational tool is only as effective as the teacher who employs it (McKenzie, 1974). Since simulation techniques require specialized skills that were not included in the graduate preparation of many nursing educators, it is necessary to develop them through practice, workshops, reading, and supplementary courses. Bevis (1978, p. 189) provides helpful ideas about how the teacher can prepare for a class using experientially based learning:

1. Formulate the student objectives (desired behavioral outcomes); make explicit the processes and information expected to be learned and the behaviors that will be outcomes.
2. Design (a) the teaching strategies, (b) possible teaching tactics, and (c) the evaluation tool.
3. Make preparatory assignment to students.
4. Require evidence of completion of assignment (optional).
5. Write a description of the learning activity for the class (if problem solving, write the problem situation).
6. Do the activity prior to requiring it of students.
7. Have a list of principles that pertain to the subject and are available for reference to ensure that appropriate content is used in the process as well as provide for comments on student activities.

Sylvester (1974) and Seidl and Dresen (1978) provide suggestions about what the teacher using a simulation activity needs to do before the simulation experience. Before and at the time of the simulation, students need information about what they are expected to accomplish; the constraints, if any, under which they must operate; and what roles and responsibilities they will have to assume. Orientation about learning outcomes directs the student's attention to what is required, thus creating a positive *set*, and motivates the student by making the relationship between the activity and learning needs explicit.

Background knowledge is important to productive involvement in simulation activities and is one factor that differentiates simulations from nonsimulation activities. With simulations, application of previously learned knowledge is required. Assignments are needed that will provide the students with guidance in obtaining necessary knowledge. Resources may include listening to lectures, completing independent learning packages, using audiovisual materials, attending workshops, and so forth. Variety is helpful so that the student can select those resources most conducive to personal learning. Guidelines for gaining desired information can also be helpful in focusing the students' attention, thus making preparation more productive.

During the Simulation Activity.　　The basic process for use of simulation is that participants are placed in a situation that involves the key variables of real-life roles, conditions, and processes in which the participants must make decisions as if they were in the actual situation. As each decision is made, consequences become known and, thus, must be considered in subsequent decisions.

If the simulation is designed as an independent activity, the teacher participates as an observer to provide feedback about behaviors or as an expert to provide clues about appropriate action. The teacher's involvement may be direct (as with one-to-one observation of a student practicing skills) or indirect (as with a videotaped sequence of a student's performance or through the interaction offered via a computer program).

Common group techniques used in simulation activities are role playing and small group discussion. Typically, a case study or problem situation is used for student analysis, consideration of alternatives and consequences, and evaluation of outcomes. The simulation may be introduced by identifying a problem (e.g., factors to consider when setting priorities) related to a particular topic, such as team leading, in order to focus the discussion in the direction desired. Common techniques used to introduce the problem situation include printed situations or videotaped sequences.

Ending the Simulation.　　One of the critical elements of simulation is that the student gains a sense of closure (i.e., completion of the learning experience). Thiagarajan and Stolovich (1978, pp. 41–42) outline four devices for achieving closure: (1) completion of a time period—establishing a time limit for the activity ahead of time; (2) achievement of a goal—making a decision; (3) completion of a task—development of a teaching plan; and (4) elimination of the competition.

The first three apply to all types of simulations, while the fourth applies to simulation games only since someone is declared a winner according to the rules of play. The authors also state that alternate devices for ending may be used. For example, the simulation can end either when a particular period of time has expired or when a specific goal or task has been accomplished. In situations where students are practicing problem-solving or manipulative skills, it is often helpful to stop the action at different points to discuss key factors, principles, or techniques of problem solving.

Postsimulation Discussion. The discussion following simulation activities is referred to as debriefing. Its purposes are "surfacing the learning" and providing closure (Bevis, 1978, p. 190). Many people believe that this is when the real learning occurs (Thiagarajan & Stolovich, 1978). Yet it is often neglected, thus limiting the amount of learning that takes place (Bevis, 1978).

Three major components of a good debriefing session are outlined by Gillespie (1973, pp. 24–27) as (1) summarization of experiences, (2) application of knowledge, and (3) integration of experiences. All three need to take place in order to review, reinforce, and clarify what the student has learned and demonstrate its application to real situations. An important part of the process is helping the student to "externalize" the problem-solving methods used. Interaction Associates (1972, p. 6) state: "By becoming conscious (aware) of the processes (strategies) he uses to resolve a problem or win a game, the student can then apply these same processes in other situations (transfer)."

One of the major techniques recommended for debriefing is that of asking questions. This can be done verbally with face-to-face contact, in written form for use during a group discussion, in written form as part of an independent learning package, or in computerized form as part of a computer program. The exact questions used will, of course, depend on the situation and the objectives of the activity. Seidl and Dresen (1978) give examples of questions that can be used in situations of conflict resolution in a complex organizational structure. Dearth and McKenzie (1975) provide examples of questions related to role-bias and its relationship to perceptions and problem solving. A few examples that can apply to any situation are given here:

1. What were your feelings at a particular moment?
2. How do values and perceptions affect decisions?
3. How does the experience relate to the objectives?
4. How can the assigned reading, etc. be applied to the experience?
5. How does the experience relate to concepts and skills to be learned?
6. How does the experience apply to other situations you have been involved in or read about?
7. What decisions were made and what were their effects?
8. What influenced the choices made?
9. What was the rationale for decisions made?
10. Did you alter your approach during the activity? If yes, why?
11. To what extent do the results reflect reality (actual problem)?
12. How can what happened be applied to real-life problems?

Finally, an important part of providing closure is a summary of major points and principles. This can be done by the teacher, the group, or individuals. As part of the summary, the student may be offered or asked to think of follow-up activities that will provide a bridge between the experience and future learning. Follow-up activities can include seeing a film, reading an article, attending a group session, or interviewing someone.

Performance in the Actual Setting. Relevance of the simulation to real-life experiences is important. A simulation that is closely followed by some real-life activity allows for application and validation of what has been learned and an integration of new skills into one's repertoire.

USING SIMULATION FOR EVALUATION

Any nursing educator will probably admit that evaluation of clinical performance is a complex and difficult process. The use of simulations for improving clinical evaluations in the health professions has been increasing (Irby & Morgan, 1974). Simulations for evaluation of clinical decision making are easier to administer than a test experience in the actual clinical setting and help to control extraneous factors that are unrelated to the test situation. Evaluation using simulation is also obviously preferable to standard paper-and-pencil tests when concentrating on psychomotor skills.

Hoban and Casberque (1978, pp. 149–150) discuss four principles that should be applied when using simulation for clinical evaluation. They are:

1. The performance (knowledge, skill, or attitude) that is expected of the student at the end of training should be specified along with the minimal acceptable level of performance the student is required to demonstrate. . . .
2. The simulation should represent reality with enough fidelity to assure face validity of the test of the student's performance. . . .
3. The simulation being used to evaluate student performance should be standardized: the simulation should produce the same kind of responses from a variety of students and provide the same feedback to students when they engage in similar activities. . . .
4. Decisions regarding the purpose of the evaluation should be made before a simulation is used. . . .

In relation to the latter, Hoban (1978) distinguishes between simulation as a diagnostic tool and simulation as a tool for certification. They represent the difference between formative and summative evaluation and place teacher and student roles and attitudes on two entirely different levels. For example, when using simulation as a diagnostic tool, the teacher functions in a supportive role in helping a student identify the direction that future work should take. This function of simulation applies particularly at the skill development stage so that students become aware of performance expectations and ways to achieve the competence needed for practice in the actual setting.

When simulation is used for certification, the role of the teacher becomes judgmental in deciding if the student has achieved the desired level of mastery. This function applies to the evaluation/testing of skills performance that is part of a course or certification procedure or to determine the level of performance of students desiring advanced placement in an educational program.

GAMES

Another technique related to simulations and simulation games in purpose and justification, but different in structure and process, is that of games, that is, games that are nonsimulation activities. The term "game" is defined as presented at the beginning of this chapter. Thus, it would involve some type of competition and a "reward" when the goal is reached. The competition may be with one's self, the game, a computer, or other people. It may not, therefore, be competition in the usual sense of the word. Many games also encourage cooperation for the achievement of group goals at the same time that they include the element of competition with others. As with simulation games, nonsimulation games can involve winners and losers, but the game can also be designed so that all participants "win" with the achievement of the stated goal, achievement of new learning, or demonstration of past learning.

Games change the traditional lecture situation into a process that is more active and motivating. As with any other strategy, they should be selected because it is thought that they are best for reaching course objectives. Games can be used with individuals, pairs, or groups. They often, but not always, require peer interaction and cooperation. They allow learning to take place in a nonthreatening, nonjudgmental atmosphere in which the student maintains more active control (Crancer & Maury-Hess, 1980).

Games can be relatively simple in design, such as simple card games, question and answer games, and adaptations of bingo. Others are much more complex, with intricate rules and procedures of play. A key factor in their success in a learning situation is that the rules are understandable and easily communicated to other people. In many instances, however, all rules do not have to be understood before the game begins, since rules and procedures can be clarified during the progress of the game.

Purposes of Educational Games

Educational games can be used to introduce a topic or concept, set up group learning situations, provide a higher degree of enjoyment with learning, serve as a medium to demonstrate knowledge and skill, provide relaxation, and serve as an alternative mechanism for evaluation and remedial work. For example, simple games involving matching items, arranging cards, or filling in crossword puzzles can be easily incorporated into an independent study package as part of the learning activity itself, for self-evaluation, or for testing. Such would be particularly appropriate to use with terminology and definitions.

In group situations, games offer an opportunity to demonstrate knowledge and skills. For example, in a team game in which members accrue points by answering specific questions, a student can gain greater self-esteem by knowing the answers and helping the team to win. It is possible, however, that self-esteem could be lowered if the student is unable to answer questions. Other learning gains may still occur, however, as a result of hearing questions and answers that stimulate recall and reinforce learning. Only a small percentage of the population does not enjoy educational games (Tansey & Unwin, 1969). This is thought to be due to a dislike of the competitive element. If this is the case, other games that focus on cooperation rather than competition can be selected.

Educational Games for Nursing

Nursing literature holds some references to the use of games, although, at times, the term is used in ways other than that defined in this chapter. For example, Davidhizar (1977) uses the term "simulation games" although it appears that the examples given are games only, with limited or no actual simulation. Sylvester (1974) refers to "management games," although examples given appear to be situations or incidents for group discussion and problem solving but without the characteristics of a game. Some authors use the terms gaming or game to refer to activities that clearly fit the definition in this chapter. Ivor (1974) uses crossword puzzles to teach medical terminology to nonnursing personnel. Pullan and Plant (1978) use a board game with cards and dice to evaluate knowledge about nursing problems. Humphrey (1974) uses a game to introduce the concept of poverty in relation to health. Rottet (1974) uses adaptations of bingo to teach coronary care nurses about cardiac arrhythmias and therapy and a matching game to assess knowledge about common methods of treatment of twenty conditions. Crancer and Maury-Hess (1980) describe the use of six games and summarize student reactions to each. Although the games described by Crancer and Maury-Hess are not commercially available, the descriptions can serve as guidelines for development. Some of the resources cited previously for design of simulations may also be helpful for the design of games (see page 43).

A brief description of several games is presented in summary form in Table 3-3. A complete example of one game is given in Appendix 2. There has been no attempt to evaluate quality or appropriateness for purposes stated. There is, rather, an attempt to include some variety of type and subject. Other commercial games can be located by referring to the references given with gamed simulations (see page 39).

LIMITATIONS AND CONCERNS

Although simulation and games have many positive features that are thought to facilitate certain types of learning, it must be stressed that they are not a cure for all problems in education. It is, therefore, impor-

Table 3-3

Examples of Nonsimulation Games Suitable for Nursing Education

Title of Game	Availability	Number of Players	Playing Time	Objectives and Description of Process of Game
Clothespin game	See Appendix 2 for complete description and directions	3 players per group; as many groups as desired	Varies	This is a game to demonstrate principles of learning in relation to discovery, modeling, and reinforcement. Allows for varying degrees of competition and reward, if desired.
I.D.-C.C.D.	Sim-Ed. College of Education University of Arizona Tucson, AZ 85721	3–5 per group; as many groups as desired	1–2 h	Assists students in identifying five common communicable diseases of childhood in relation to common and medical terminology, incubation periods, communicability periods, symptomology. Prior preparation is required. Positive and negative reinforcement are used (Sim-Ed, 1978).
Word games, Vols. 1 and 2	American Journal of Nursing Co. Educational Services Division New York, NY 10019	Individual	Varies	Contains vocabulary games, including crossword puzzles, word searches, and word scrambles. Goal is improvement of vocabulary and spelling skills.
Bingo I and Bingo II	John Wiley & Sons 605 Third Avenue New York, NY 10158	3–9	Varies	Competitive games that emphasize rapid thinking and recall. Focus is on reinforcement and retention of learning. Bingo I requires knowledge of drug classifications. Bingo II requires knowledge of diagnostic tests and respiratory drugs (Wolf & Duffy, 1979).
Nutrition game	Graphics Co. P.O. Box 331 Urbana, IL 61801	2–6	1–2 h	Designed to increase knowledge about nutrients, food costs, and health. Uses cards with common foods as well as penalty cards, bonus cards, and play money (Huebner-Zappia, undated).
Downer roulette	Spinco Medical Corp. Box 8113 Waco, TX 76710	Any	½–1 h	Participants spin a roulette wheel. Final score depends on whether alcohol has been mixed with other "downers." Possible game results range from relaxed, to coma, to death (Huebner-Zappia, undated).

tant to be aware of some of the potential limitations or problems that can be associated with simulation and games. The following are key points that have been summarized from several resources (Seidl & Dresen, 1978; Wolf & Duffy, 1979; Pearson, 1975; Thiagarajan & Stolovich, 1978):

1. When too much emphasis is placed on the details of the activity rather than on the process, when too much emphasis is placed on competition, or when students do not associate enjoyable activities with learning, students can be left with a lack of sense of learning.
2. When there is oversimplification of reality, students can be led into improper learning or a mistaken illusion of understanding.
3. When activities are performed exclusively in a group or exclusively alone, the needs of all students may not be met.
4. When there is inadequate debriefing to externalize learning, when there is a lack of follow-up application, or when students are distracted by unrelated events or personal frustrations, learning can be incomplete.
5. When the model for reality is biased, there can be an improper manipulation of attitudes and values.
6. When emotions are involved, some students can become overly intense or anxious.
7. The amount of time and effort required to develop simulations and games reduces their likelihood of cost-effectiveness in comparison with traditional methods.
8. Teachers who are tradition bound may have difficulty in dealing with the loss of control over students, the stringent requirements of process teaching, the increased level of activity in the classroom, and the use of seemingly "frivolous" methods for serious purposes.

These limitations and problems can be dealt with somewhat by the systematic development of the activity, careful selection and use of simulation and games for specific purposes, thorough preplanning by the teacher, and adequate inservice training and teacher training in the use of nontraditional methods.

SUMMARY

This chapter has dealt with simulation and games as they can be applied to nursing education. There has been a particular attempt made to clarify definitions of terms. Claims about potential learning benefits and research findings about effectiveness have been presented. Although empirical evidence to support effectiveness for learning is limited, various learning theories justify the use of simulation and games among other strategies. Simulation types and examples, purposes, and procedures for use, along with purposes and examples of games for nursing, have been discussed. The chapter ends with a listing of limitations and concerns and possible ways of dealing with them.

APPENDIX 1
SAMPLE SIMULATION GAME: HERE COMES THE JUDGE*

Purpose

To facilitate participation in a group endeavor to solve simulated nursing problems.

Description

A game called "Here Comes the Judge" employs the team concept and intergroup cooperation to beat the other team. Each group solves a specific given problem about a topic selected by the teacher. The groups go through all phases of the problem-solving process; they carefully document each alternative that might be an acceptable intervention, select an intervention, and justify the intervention selection with sound documentation. One team presents the problem as they solved it going through each stage. The challengers must catch them out—find and prove the flaws. In cases of impasse a group of judges makes decisions about who wins the point.

Points accumulate, and the winning group is rewarded.

Objectives

This game is contrived so that to reach the established goal the participant will:

1. Gather, organize, document, and assimilate information collected by the participants.
2. Critically choose the information and predictive principles appropriate to specific problems.
3. Utilize data in the appropriate facets of problem solving.

*From Bevis, E. O. *Curriculum building in nursing* (2nd ed.). St. Louis: Mosby, 1978, pp. 187–188. Used by permission.

4. Participate in a mutually accountable way in a group problem-solving endeavor.
5. Use other members of the group for information, validation, feedback, negotiation, and judgment.
6. Encourage communications, peer support, evaluation, and critiquing of the authoritative resources cited and question validity of resources by citing authoritative opposing views.
7. Utilize the problem-solving strengths of all members of the group by varying player roles and group composition.

Rules

The class is divided into three basic groups:

1. The group presenting (usually 3 to 5 students).
2. The group who have the first right of challenge (usually 3 to 5 students).
3. The group of judges who arbitrate challenges and rebuttals and award the decision to the group who best substantiate their statements. The awards are made in points, and the judges keep score. If the groups wish to award prizes, they may determine what these are to be—losers buy Cokes, and so forth.
4. If the class is larger than 15 to 18 students, the students not immediately involved in one of the three groups have the privilege of challenging any decision after it has been made and before the next phase of problem solving continues; however, their challenge must be substantiated as above. If in the opinion of the judges this group makes their challenge, they collect the point.

Procedure of Play

The game may be used for the solving of a whole problem or for any selected part of problem solving, that is, problem identification phase, problem data phase, or decision phase. The game can be spread over several class periods or contained in one period. Several class periods permit additional research by enthusiastic players. Books and so forth are permitted in class.

1. Statements on transparencies or on butcher paper may be prepared ahead of time or as part of the class.
2. A member of the presenting group is chosen by that group to act as moderator for the group. However, it is the responsibility of all the presenting members to coach and strengthen the group's presentation, that is, to assume responsibility for making as valid and strong a case as possible for their portion of solving a problem.
3. The presenting group presents the whole problem briefly. This gives the players an overview and prevents challenging material that is covered later. During this overall presentation, challenge groups can take notes on incor-

rect, omitted, or extraneous material for use during the challenge part of the game.

4. Points are awarded by the judges as follows:
   a. The presenting group gets 1 point for correct and accepted presented material.
   b. The group citing data or material omitted by the presenting group collects 1 point for each concept area accepted by the judges as essential omitted material.
   c. Challenged material is arbitrated by the judges, and the group who are adjudged as correct win 1 point. If the presenting group are deemed correct they are awarded 1 point for being incorrectly challenged; if the challenge group are deemed correct, they are awarded 1 point for being proper in their challenge.
   d. Material that is included by the presenting group that is challenged for being extraneous, inappropriate, tangential, or unnecessary to the solution of the problem can be awarded a point for the winning group in the same way.

APPENDIX 2
SAMPLE NONSIMULATION GAME: CLOTHESPIN
GAME TO LEARN ABOUT LEARNING*

Objectives

At the end of this activity you will be able to:

1. State the difference in discovery learning and modeling.
2. Compare the differences in time needed to learn a task among (a) those using exploration and discovery learning techniques, (b) those using modeling techniques, and (c) those who have the benefit of practice.
3. Identify the role of reinforcement in learning and name some of the forms that reinforcement takes.
4. List learning propositions that can be derived from this activity.

Directions

1. Divide into groups of three players.
2. Designate one person as discovery learner, one person as modeling learner, and one person as timer-recorder.

*From Bevis, E. O. *Curriculum building in nursing* (2nd ed.). St. Louis: Mosby, 1978, pp. 188–189. Used by permission.

3. Take six wooden pieces and three metal pieces from the clothespin box.

4. Give two wooden pieces and one metal piece to both the discovery learner and the modeling learner.

5. The discovery learner must put the clothespin together without prompting or guidance from the other members of the group.

6. The timer times, in seconds, how long it takes the discovery learner to complete the task.

7. The timer and the modeling learner smile, nod, encourage, clap, cheer, or do anything else they think will encourage and reinforce the discovery learner while he is doing his task as long as they think he is moving in the direction that will lead to success. They may not offer him any advice or directions.

8. The timer marks down the time used by the discovery learner in completing his task.

9. The modeling learner places the clothespin that is now back together in front of him. Using it as a model and having observed the discovery learner complete the task, the modeling learner proceeds to put the second clothespin together.

10. The timer again times the operation and records the time in seconds. The difference in the two times is calculated.

11. The discovery learner and the timer use the same reinforcing tactics listed in item 7 to encourage and reinforce the modeling learner.

12. The discovery learner takes the remaining two pieces of wood and one wire and puts the clothespin together. He can look at the clothespins that are put together, if he chooses. Reinforcing behaviors are again used by the other group members.

13. The timer again times the discovery learner and records the time as "practice number 2."

14. Someone collects the times, averages them, and puts the findings on the blackboard.

15. Each group uses assigned texts, class notes, any other available resources and experiences, feelings and observations made during the activity to list learning propositions they saw enacted or experienced while participating.

16. The class may or may not wish to award a prize to the group identifying the most nearly complete and accurate list of learning propositions that they saw in actual operation during the activity.

4

Developing
Psychomotor Skills

Astronauts are rocketed into space and sent on journeys around the earth only after they have mastered all the skills essential for successful flight. Many of these skills are complex psychomotor skills that require hours of practice and rehearsal to ensure mastery. Each planned movement is carried out with accuracy and efficiency, because there is no place for human error or hesitancy at the controls of a spacecraft. In other words, only those who have reached complete mastery of the art and science of space flight are sent aloft.

In basic nursing education programs, students are prepared to enter the profession with many beginning skills. The novice is not expected to have mastered all of the skills embodied in practice before embarking into the work setting.

The acquisition of skills has long been the primary desire of nursing students during their educational programs (Paynich, 1971). Recently, strong interest in this area has been displayed by new graduates, nursing service employers, and faculties of nursing schools (Collins & Joel, 1971; Benner & Benner, 1979). Nursing service settings have developed programs that focus on the skill development and practice needs of the beginning nurse (Atwood, 1979).

This chapter was written by Sharon Eaton, R.N., M.S., Assistant Professor of Nursing, University of San Francisco, California, and Grace Davis, R.N., M.A., Director, Department of Education and Training, Children's Hospital, San Francisco, California.

LEVELS OF PERFORMANCE

Psychomotor skills are often a major component of procedure or skill lists used to determine levels of performance of the recent graduate. Skills lists are commonly used as guides for planning experiences that offer practice in those nursing procedures essential to patient care. The level of competence of students or novice nurses is often judged by the degree to which they can smoothly and efficiently perform nursing procedures. Teachers of nurses play a vital role in helping learners acquire the skills needed for practice. This chapter discusses the area of psychomotor skill learning, its importance in the practice of nursing, and implications for teachers.

Psychomotor skills are described by Richardson (1969) as manipulative skills that require the learner to perceive and coordinate sensory stimuli to complete purposeful movements. Children learn many psychomotor skills essential to the development of independence and survival in the world around them. Adults continue to learn and develop psychomotor skills to help them adapt to the demands of the reality-based work world.

Nursing schools graduate students who are beginning practitioners. Practice and experience are required before the beginner can be expected to reach a high level of competence in the art and science of nursing. The nursing literature (Lewis, E. P., 1971; Gudmundsen, 1975) is filled with pleas for a return of the "art" to nursing. One component of this art is the smooth performance of procedures and the dexterous handling of equipment.

COMPONENTS OF PSYCHOMOTOR LEARNING

To understand the nature of psychomotor learning, a brief review of the theories that guide this area of learning is in order.

Bloom (1956) described the importance of the psychomotor area of learning as one of the three learning domains—cognitive, affective, and psychomotor. He stated that teachers had responsibilities for writing objectives and planning learning activities to meet the objectives of each of the three domains. Nursing school curricula reflect the attention given to each of these domains as teachers plan learning goals for their students.

Because psychomotor performance involves observable behavior, it has been especially appealing to behaviorists. Robert Gagné focused on the stimulus-response (S-R) theory to outline the conditions for chaining that occurred in the carrying out of a skill. The six conditions Gagné (1965; 1974) identified are:

1. Each S-R connection must have been previously learned (e.g., to open a locked door a person must be able to identify the upright position of the key, insert it in the lock, turn it, and push the door open).
2. The steps, or links, in the chain must be performed in the proper order. This could be taught either by demonstrating the proper sequence and then inviting the learner to perform, or by using verbal instructions as prompts (e.g., "All right, now that you have the key in the lock, turn it, and then push the door open").
3. The individual steps must be performed in close succession to establish the chain.
4. Repetition is usually necessary if the act is to be performed easily and efficiently, since it often takes several tries to smooth out clumsy and superfluous movements.
5. The terminal step, or link, must result in success, which provides reinforcement (e.g., the door must open).
6. Once a motor skill has been learned, it can be generalized (e.g., the technique for opening one lock can be applied to opening a slightly different one). However, it may be necessary to teach the student to discriminate if there is a significant difference in the second act (e.g., opening a lock by turning the key counterclockwise).

To develop teaching methods for learning complex psychomotor skills, the teacher analyzes the skill and divides it into its parts or subskills. The subskills are placed in logical order. The learner sees the total psychomotor skill demonstrated, then each subskill is identified and demonstrated in sequence.

Supervised practice periods are provided immediately following the demonstration. As learners practice, the teacher provides verbal guidance and reinforcement. Learners carry out the complete skill unassisted. The teacher might identify similarities between skills that learners had previously mastered and new psychomotor skills. The teacher needs to be alert for any conditions within the practice setting that might interfere with learning (fatigue of learner, noisy environment, etc.).

Skinner (1968) used the phrase "movement duplication" to describe learning motor skills. He said that modeling was the first and vital step in the learning of a motor skill. The aim of modeling was to make the behaviors conspicuous to the learner. Later, the learner might practice in front of a mirror or be recorded on videotape to become his own model. Practice was a necessary component of duplication as Skinner described it.

Simpson (1966) described another dimension in the acquisition of a psychomotor skill. She described the following mental aspects of skill acquisition:

Perception is a crucial beginning step in performing a motor act. It is the process of sensory input, cue selection, and translation. The learner places, in priority order, sensory stimulation and environmental cues and relates these to the action in performing a motor act. For example, when a nurse changes a child's bottle of intravenous solution, the process of perception occurs. The nurse observes and handles the bottle and tubing, is sensitive to the child's needs for reassurance and the parents' needs for information, and recalls the principles of aseptic technique learned in the past.

Readiness, or *set,* occurs when the learner has developed mental, physical, and emotional readiness to perform the actions. In other words, learners are able to call upon mental pictures of themselves beginning the action, having the physical and physiological capabilities to complete the action, and are psychologically ready to try. Simpson's taxonomy (1966) continues with descriptions of performance responses.

Guided response is discussed as an early step in skill development. During this phase, learners imitate actions they have seen demonstrated. With the cueing of the teacher and by trial and error, learners achieve appropriate responses.

Mechanism includes learned responses that become habitual. Learners now have confidence and some skill in performing procedures.

Complex overt response is described as the final level in psychomotor skill acquisition. Uncertainty has been resolved; performance is smooth, precise, free from hesitancy, and has become automatic.

In addition to the process of teaching psychomotor skills as described by these theorists, attention needs to be focused on other aspects of the teaching-learning process. Richardson (1969) has described in detail the use of visualization as an important factor in improving skills performance. He described how learners were able to improve their skills in dart throwing, high jumping, and hooping baskets by simply carrying out those motions in their mind's eye. Students simply sat in the classroom, closed their eyes, and "saw" themselves performing these acts successfully. Athletic coaches emphasize and assist their students in developing skills of visualization to improve skill performance and develop internal readiness.

TEACHING PSYCHOMOTOR SKILLS

To apply the above theories to nursing education, the teacher starts by describing why and how each specific psychomotor skill fits into the total practice of art of nursing. The needs for safety of practice and assurance of quality care for people are among the most important reasons. This explanation forms the basis on which the teacher then plans experiences for the learner.

The *demonstration phase* of teaching deserves careful attention. The initial demonstration should be smooth, skilled, and successful. All learners should be able to see and hear clearly. In a large group when intricate hand movements are being demonstrated, a video camera might be focused on the demonstration with monitors placed throughout the room so that learners are able to watch movements on a television screen.

It is during the step-by-step demonstration that Skinner's (1968) suggestions of exaggerating movement and slowing down action are helpful. To illustrate this process, a skill foreign to many but an enjoyable one—that of a basic tap dance step—could be chosen. The dance step is demonstrated on a tabletop where all learners can hear the count and see the foot tapping out each of the five components of the step. The demonstration is repeated several times, starting with one foot and then the other foot, until all the learners in the room are tapping in time. At the end of 5 minutes, all learners are able to imitate the five components of the step. Smooth, skilled imitation or mastery is not the aim of this exercise, but some learners with prior dance experience may be able to perform skillfully. This exercise combines the phases of demonstration and guided practice. Learners receive positive verbal reinforcement as they imitate each component of the exercise. As is often the case, those who learn quickly help others until the whole group learns the tap step.

If equipment is used during a demonstration, the individual parts should be identified by name and function. This is most effectively done after the initial total demonstration has been completed and repeated demonstrations begun.

The expert practitioner is not always the best person to demonstrate complex psychomotor skills. Learners may feel overwhelmed, put down, and hesitant to try a new procedure if teachers are tempted to "show off" expert skills in the demonstration phase. Another cautionary note about the use of experts to demonstrate skills is offered by Dreyfus and Dreyfus (1981). They describe "experts" as those who have incorporated each of the factors (steps) of the skill into their performance to the extent that they can no longer identify the factors or steps. In the demonstration phase, it is important that the steps be identified clearly for the learner.

The next phase in learning psychomotor skills is *guided practice*. Some helpful hints for teachers to consider during this phase are:

1. Learners need to explore and manipulate equipment as soon as possible after the demonstration. They need the tactile experience in order to diffuse anxiety that might be generated about handling equipment. Learners are encouraged to explore materials using all their senses and to handle equipment with their eyes shut so that kinesthetic feelings are aroused. Many adult learners are self-conscious about trying new psychomotor skills. They worry about looking foolish and making errors. It is crucial that the learning environment be made warm and accepting, inviting the learners to try things, take risks, and experiment.

2. Individual differences are important variables in learning psychomotor skills. Some of the differences might be related to manual dexterity, attitude, motivation, confidence, kinesthetic awareness, intelligence, or age of the learners. In planning learning experiences, these factors must be considered.

3. Practice periods vary for individual learners and take a variety of forms. Complexity of the psychomotor skill determines the amount and type of practice required to learn the skill. Such activities as knitting or needlework have been used to develop fine motor movements and finger flexibility.

4. Feedback on performance during the practice phase is vital to reinforce correct behaviors and eliminate errors. Peer groups are useful for analyzing performance and providing immediate feedback. Videotaping can be used effectively by learners to critique their own performance during this stage.

5. When a learner is stuck at one step of the performance and consistently errs, it may be helpful to have the learner repeat the error over and over to make it very visual and bring awareness of the error to a conscious level. The teacher may, if done with good humor, demonstrate and exaggerate the error so that the learner sees and acknowledges it. It is wise to remember that an adult learner is fragile when frustrated. In this self-centered state, the learner may overreact to less-than-tender methods of correction.

6. Teachers should be aware of left-handed learners and make provisions for them. These learners may find it helpful to face the teacher and mirror the movements. Right handed learners may prefer to

imitate the teacher's movements by standing beside the teacher and facing in the same direction.

7. Teachers should remain silent except to offer positive cues and give encouragement to learners as they perform each step. Beginners who have no basis on which to evaluate their own performance need feedback when they complete each step. Teachers must avoid the temptation to take the learners' hands and guide the performance, because learners need to perform movements independently. If teachers point out similarities between new and previously learned skills, it helps learners transfer information to new situations. For example, there are similarities between handling a bulb syringe to perform an irrigation and the manipulation of a disposable syringe to administer a medication.

8. It may be helpful if teachers share personal examples of their own ineptitude as they initially learned skills. It may comfort struggling learners to know that others had problems in the beginning. However, learners tend to be self-centered in skill acquisition, so references to the experiences of others should be limited.

Simulation experiences are frequently used during the guided practice phase. Pilots who are learning to fly an airplane are taught in a simulated environment. They learn flight maneuvers in a model long before they enter the cockpit of the actual aircraft. Similarly, nursing programs have simulated environments in which learners can manipulate models and equipment free from the pressures of the actual situation (Infante, 1981).

Some educators question the value of simulated experiences. Thorndike warned in the 1930s (Bugelski, 1971) that there might not be such a thing as transfer learning. Skills are learned strictly in the situational context presented and need to be relearned in any other context. Montag (1951) also questioned the transfer value of simulated experiences and placed nursing students directly in the clinical area to learn basic skills. Whether or not simulated experiences accelerate skill acquisition may be still in question, but learners report feeling more adept when they practice in a skills laboratory. If they perceive themselves to be more skilled, perhaps this perception enables them to perform with more confidence, less hesitancy, and increased skill.

The final stage in the development of a psychomotor skill is *mastery*. Mastery performance is skilled, smooth, dexterous, efficient, and is adapted to incorporate cues from the current situation. Mastery is rarely accomplished in the student phase of learning and is the accomplishment of very few. Acceptable levels of performance of psychomotor skills are most often not at a mastery level.

Once attained, the maintenance of mastery level of achievement requires continued practice. One component of practice at this level is mental rehearsal. For example, musicians, golfers, athletes, and others prepare themselves for performances by first visualizing themselves in action and performing at peak level. To use a nursing example, nurses who have mastered the dialysis procedure report the value of time spent rehearsing the procedure verbally and visually before they begin the procedure with a patient.

SUMMARY

Improving the performance of psychomotor skills is one of the solutions to returning the "art" to nursing. The development of psychomotor skills is complex, and examples from the fields of art, aviation, athletics, and nursing can illustrate the process of skill acquisition. Consideration of the developmental process should be a guide for those involved in teaching skills and evaluating performance.

Teaching methods, such as visualization, cueing, and other techniques, facilitate skill acquisition.

5

Asking Questions

Teachers ask students questions for a variety of reasons. They may wish to find out what a student already knows about a given subject or situation, or they may wish to stimulate interest in a new topic. Teachers may use questions as a stimulus variation from lecturing. Or, teachers may utilize questions as feedback to determine if students have already grasped the major points under consideration. Questions, when skillfully asked, help students to see relationships and link the unknown to the known. In addition, questioning permits student and teacher to explore ideas together. The art of questioning, more than any other single teaching skill, can assist teachers in conveying their interest, enthusiasm, and continued pursuit of learning.

What teachers need to give and what they need to ask form an important facet of teaching strategies (Taba, 1967). If the development of students' autonomy in thinking is an important objective, the "seeking" functions of teaching assume greater importance than those of "giving." In order for students to develop concepts by their own efforts, teachers must become adroit guiders of the heuristic process.

Basically, there are three kinds of questions—factual or descriptive, clarifying, and higher order.

FACTUAL OR DESCRIPTIVE QUESTIONS

Factual questions include those that can be answered from either memory or by description. Factual questions are elicited by such words as:

who, what, when, or *where.* For a factual question, the student is asked to recall information previously acquired. Many facts are important because they provide the building blocks for concepts and generalizations. The following are examples of factual questions:

1. "What is the normal white blood cell count?"
2. "What is the normal range of blood pressure?"
3. "Who is eligible for welfare in our country?"

Descriptive questions, although more complicated than factual questions, require that students respond from either memory or simple descriptive statements. They, too, deal mostly with facts. Descriptive questions differ from factual questions in that the student is required to organize thoughts in a logical relationship and to respond with a longer answer than the straight-forward response of the factual question. Examples of descriptive questions are:

1. "What are differences in the symptoms of a patient in diabetic coma and in insulin shock?"
2. "Who is eligible for medicare and medicaid?"
3. "What does Satir mean when she calls one member of the family the 'identified patient'?"

CLARIFYING QUESTIONS

The second type of question is the clarifying question. Clarifying requires that teachers ask questions that help students to go beyond a superficial response. This can be done in five ways (Far Western Laboratory for Educational Research and Development, 1969):

1. *Asking questions for more information and/or more meaning*
   The teacher seeks additional clarification from the student. Examples of questions that might be asked are:
   A. "I don't quite understand what you mean."
   B. "Tell us more about the point you just made."
   C. "What do you mean by the term _____?"
2. *Requiring student to justify response*
   Here the teacher wants to be certain the student really understands the point just made in order to increase the student's critical awareness. Such questions designed to assist the student are:
   A. "What are the assumptions you are making?"

   B. "What are your reasons for thinking this is so?"

   C. "Suppose you were debating your point of view with an opponent. What points might your opponent bring out?"

3. *Refocusing the student's attention on a related issue*
The teacher may wish to assist students to clarify a different, but related, issue in order to foster transfer. Examples of refocusing questions include:

   A. "What are the implications of this discussion for patients who are not hospitalized?"

   B. "How does this relate to . . . ?"

   C. "How does John's response relate to Joan's?"

4. *Prompting the student*
If the students are unable to determine relationships for themselves, a hint from the teacher may assist them. Examples of prompting questions include:

TEACHER: "Mary, you have stated that your nursing care plan for Mrs. Smith included special skin care. What is the reason?"

MARY: "Her skin is edematous. This requires special care."

TEACHER: "That's very true. What are some of the complications that can occur when excess fluid is retained in the tissue?"

MARY: "Edema predisposes to infection."

TEACHER: "Right! Any special reason why this happens?"

MARY: "Well, I don't know."

TEACHER: "What might there be about edema that predisposes to infection?"

MARY: "Oh, I see. It probably is a good culture media for infection."

TEACHER: "And what might some other complications be?"

5. *Redirecting the question*
This is a technique designed to broaden the participation of other students in a clarifying session by changing the interaction from the teacher and one student to the teacher and other students. An example of redirecting is:

TEACHER: "Mary, you have stated that Mrs. Smith complained of thirst following her surgery. What might be the reason for this symptom?"

MARY: "She was given preoperative medications that decreased her fluid production."

TEACHER: "That's one possible reason. Paul, what might be other plausible reasons?"

Other techniques could include asking other students why they agreed or disagreed with a student's response.

HIGHER-ORDER QUESTIONS

The third type of questions is called higher-order questions. These include those questions that cannot be answered simply from memory or perception. Higher-order questions prod students to think beyond the facts, sequences, descriptions, or set of circumstances. They help students to establish relationships, compare and contrast concepts and principles, make inferences, see causes and effects, and find rules and principles rather than merely define them. Furthermore, they help students to use ideas freely and critically.

The word "why" is frequently used in higher-order questions. "Why" questions frequently require the student to go beyond the factual or descriptive answer by generalizing, inferring, classifying, or concluding. However, the mere use of the word "why" in a question does not necessarily guarantee that such a question is a higher-order question. For example, asking a student "Why does blood pressure elevate when blood vessels are constricted?" is a straightforward factual question if the student need only repeat what has been read in a textbook or previously learned. Were the student required to figure out the answer, it would be a higher-order question. Depending on the student's previous experiences, what may be a factual question for one student may be a higher-order question for the other.

Higher-order questions perform three specific functions:

1. *Seeking evaluation*
   Evaluative questions have no "right" answer but deal with matters of judgment, value, and choice. In order to arrive at an answer, students must set up standards and measure the idea at hand against such a standard. An example of such a question would be:
   "Should every family have a guaranteed minimum income?"
2. *Seeking inferences*
   An inference is an idea or conclusion following from a set of facts or a premise. These questions may be used when the teacher wishes students to relate something newly learned to something previously learned. They may be used to derive a reason or motive from a set of circumstances. An example of a question designed to foster inference is:

percent of the total number of questions asked by the teachers and students during these conferences. Based on their findings, these investigators pose an important question to all nursing faculty: are nursing instructors who ask low level questions justified in expecting their students to develop high level skills, such as those involved in the processes of analyzing, synthesizing, or evaluating?

In another study, Craig and Page (1981) were interested in finding out if the level of questions asked by nursing instructors could be improved by the use of a teaching module specifically developed to provide the information and practice necessary to classify, generate, and evaluate questions in terms of Bloom's (1956) work. Learning activities designed to meet these higher objectives included the classification, generation, and analysis of questions asked during an instructor's recorded postclinical conference with students. Using a pretest-posttest control group design, these investigators found that the experimental group exposed to the self-instructional module asked a greater percentage of higher-level questions than did the control group. These investigators believe that their study supports the conclusion that nursing faculty can increase the percentage of higher-level questions asked when they have inservice education in the instructional skills needed to conduct postclinical conferences. They also concluded from their study that whereas the nursing knowledge and expertise of the instructors was evident, many conferences consisted of a student recital of the tasks performed during the clinical experiences as well as a description of a patient's diagnosis, medications, and treatment. They point out that such enumeration of data really does little to foster the cognitive processes required for effective problem solving needed for the practice of nursing.

Gall (1970) raises some important questions about teacher behaviors in regard to questioning strategies. Essentially, he points out that given the importance of questions in teaching, researchers still do not know much about them. He asks two exceedingly important questions: (1) What educational objectives can questions help students to achieve? and (2) What are the criteria of an effective question and how can effective questions be identified? He also cautions that questions asked by an instructor should not be viewed as an end in themselves, but rather as a means to an end—producing desired changes in student behavior.

In his discussion about questioning behaviors, Gall (1970) raises another issue of great importance to nursing instructors. He states that the types of questions that students ask should be of great interest to instructors. For example, in introducing a new topic, students should be asked what they believe they need to know. This is of utmost importance for nursing students as they prepare for clinical experiences. The instructor who desires to develop inquiry attitudes in students will foster question-asking skills in students and then will provide reinforcement for such behaviors.

Higher-order questions are difficult for the teacher as well as for the student. They require an excellent grasp of the objectives to be achieved and knowledge beyond the given facts for both teacher and student. However, the positive reinforcement from students who are stimulated beyond the usual responses should help the teacher to become motivated to practice this technique.

SEQUENCING QUESTIONS

The sequencing of questions is of specific importance in planning a questioning strategy. If higher-order questions are asked before students have the specific information or recall required to respond to the questions, they, or the teacher, may become frustrated and discouraged. The following represents a specific questioning strategy utilizing all types of questions previously discussed:

1. *Eliciting facts or conditions*
   "What is happening?"
   "How does it happen?"
   "When does it happen?"
   "Where does it happen?"

2. *Eliciting explanations or comparisons*
   "Why does this happen?"
   "What are the variations? Why?"
   "Why do you find it so?"

3. *Clarifying for generalizations and consequences*
   "What does this mean?"
   "What does it accomplish?"
   "How do you explain it?"
   "In what other situations would it apply?"

It is not necessary to follow the above sequence in order. Teachers may begin asking questions at the second, or even the third, level. Should students not be able to respond to a higher-level question, the teacher may find it desirable to ask questions to elicit lower-level response and then ask the higher-level type of questions.

Prior to a questioning strategy, it is necessary that the teacher *set the focus*. This establishes both the topic to be discussed and the particular cognitive operation to be performed. If this is not clearly done, the students will tend to indulge in associative thinking and branch off to some word or phrase and elaborate tangentially, which can lead to topics not relevant to the discussion. Focused questions can be open-ended, permitting alternative answers, or closed, limiting responses to one "right" answer. Asking, for example, what is the daily requirement of calcium leads to one right answer. However, if the teacher asks for the reasons some persons have a calcium deficiency, this will lead to a variety of speculations and additional use of knowledge.

Questions such as "What constitutes good care of a patient in traction?" will foster training in the arbitrary evaluation of information and may develop unproductive modes of thinking in students. Such a question assumes that one can judge without a criterion. Students have two alternatives. They can guess what the teacher wants or they can try to remember what the book says. A focused question would include the criteria. For example: "How would you provide countertraction for a patient in Buck's traction?"

The impact of questioning lies not in its single acts, but in the manner in which the skilled teacher is able to combine the types of questions into a pattern. These include the particular combination of focusing, extending, and lifting from one level to another; the length of time spent on a particular operation; how the functions of giving and seeking are distributed; and the way in which the intake of information is alternated with the processing, transforming, and synthesizing of information.

One final word about questioning. Note how attorneys phrase questions. They ask one question at a time. Saying to a student in the clinical area, "What medication are you giving; what is its dose; for what is it given; and what are the side effects?" is an overloaded question, to put it mildly. It is difficult to think and listen at the same time. Therefore, by asking one part of a question at one time, it helps the student to sort out parts of a question.

SUMMARY

Questioning techniques are used for a variety of reasons. These include finding out what a student already knows about a subject or situation, as a feedback mechanism, or to develop autonomy in thinking. Questioning permits students and teachers to explore ideas together.

6

Creating Set

The term *set* refers to the response system that predisposes an individual to view and approach a problem in a predetermined manner. Hyman (1964) defines set as an attitude of mind and an organizer of information. Those actions leading to the stimulation or evoking of a set in a learner are referred as as *set induction* in learning psychology. The concept of preinstructional procedures, or set induction, comes from the research on learning indicating that activities preceding a learning task will influence the outcome of that task. Some instructional sets promote learning superior to others for certain specified learning goals.

Set induction provides a motivational aspect to learning. De Cecco and Crawford (1974) have identified three concepts—arousal, expectancy, and incentives—as major factors that account for motivation. These three concepts also point the way toward helping the instructor develop techniques to guide the student toward being motivated to learn.

AROUSAL

The arousal function is the instructor's effort toward maintaining the student's interest in learning. It involves the continuing responsibility to guard against boredom during learning. It involves actively involving the student in the learning process. By providing a certain measure of freedom to wander from one aspect to another in order to allow stu-

75

dents to discover relationships and meanings, the instructor creates an environment that fosters excitement. In such an environment, curiosity, exploration, and discovery will prevail. This is the environment in which the students find it fun and invigorating to learn and safe to make mistakes.

EXPECTANCY

The expectancy function of the teacher requires that learning objectives be described specifically for the student in terms of what the student will be able to do and know when a particular class, unit, project, or experience has been completed. Statements of instructional objectives should be concrete enough for the student to know the outcome that the teacher expects. A specific objective focuses the learner and gives promise that something new will be achieved. De Cecco and Crawford (1974) point out that, unfortunately, students become accustomed to abstract statements of instructional goals and have learned from past experiences that they can ignore them without harmful consequences. An example of a concrete statement to guide the learner is, "At the completion of today's class on the concept of *anxiety* you will be able to identify several differing behaviors of patients who exhibit anxiety." The instructor should continue by giving several contrasting examples of patient behaviors, such as the patient who talks incessantly and rings for the nurse constantly and the patient who is withdrawn and emotionally immobilized. By asking the students which example illustrates the concept *anxiety* more fully, the students can grasp the full range of the behaviors that illustrate the concept, and they are also set toward the learning goal.

INCENTIVE

The incentive factor closely relates to positive reinforcement as discussed in Chapter 1. Promising to provide feedback to students and developing checkpoints and standards for assessing their own achievement, and a positive approach toward the learning process all provide reassurance to students.

Set induction also helps students to build a cognitive bridge from what preceded to what will follow in the instructional sequence. The creative use of set induction provides the teacher with tools to help students to see the relevance of the learning experience. The activities for which set induction is particularly appropriate are:

1. *At the beginning of a course*
   The first introduction can help students to become excited about the learning experience to follow, interact readily and enthusiastically with the teacher, and explore the literature and other resources with meaningful purpose.

2. *Before classroom discussion*
   Precueing students about the expectations of the discussion will frequently prevent the wasting of time caused when students do not really understand the purpose of the discussion.

3. *Preceding a new clinical experience*
   Here the relieving of the anxiety of the unknown, the reassurance that the experience to follow is one for which the student has been prepared, and the linking of this experience with previous experiences are essential.

4. *Making an assignment*
   A set designed to increase attention to the task tends to increase the desire of the student to complete the assignment for intrinsic motivation and curiosity rather than completion merely to meet requirements to achieve a grade.

INFLUENCE OF SET

Every person has experienced set. If we are told that a given speaker is an expert, we tend to regard what the speaker says with more credibility. If we are led to believe that a given task is difficult, then we will find it so. If we are helped to see the relevance of a task, we will find the learning more meaningful and will be motivated to learn.

Set, then, predisposes us to view and approach a situation in a given way. An example of the influence of set in solving problems was experimentally illustrated by Luchins (1942). He gave his subjects, who ranged from elementary school pupils to graduate students, jars of differing sizes and instructed them to obtain a specified amount of water by using only the measures of the jars available. He substituted both different jars and amounts of water to be obtained for a series of problems. For the first problem he asked the subjects to obtain 20 quarts of water by using a 29-quart jar and a 3-quart jar. He showed the subjects how this could be accomplished by filling the 29-quart jar and then filling the 3-quart jar three times. Similarly, in order to get 100 quarts from a 127-quart jar, a 21-quart jar and a 3-quart jar, the subjects would need to fill the 127-quart jar, pour off 21 quarts, leaving 106 quarts and then pour off 3 quarts two times to achieve 100 quarts. After several such examples involving three different sizes of jars, Luchins asked his subjects to obtain 20 quarts from a 23-quart jar, a 49-quart jar and a 3-quart jar. A significant number of his subjects continued to utilize the three jar technique, even when the simple solution involved merely pouring off three quarts into the 3-quart jar from the 23-quart jar. Thus, Luchins concluded that the subjects were under the influence of a predisposing way of solving the problem.

Another simple example of how set influences us is to ask persons to draw four lines connecting all of the nine dots below without tracing back or lifting the pencil from the paper.

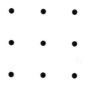

It is interesting to note that most individuals attempt to solve the problem by drawing lines *within* the confines of the nine dots. The solution lies in going beyond the dots, as below:

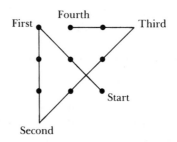

Predisposition tends to tell us to confine our solutions to previously learned tasks rather than find new or creative solutions. Both of the examples just discussed demonstrate what is referred to as "functional fixedness." The problem solver has been using information from one situation to the next when it will not operate successfully for the new situation. One simple example of "functional fixedness" is using an item for a single purpose when it may have several. A rubber ball is something to be thrown, and it also may provide excellent squeezing exercise for the hand.

The principles of the two examples just discussed are well illustrated in a study by Tuckman, Henkelman, O'Shaughnessy, and Cole (1967). They wanted to find out the effects of appropriate and inappropriate practice experiences on students' approaches to arithmetic problems.

Three short experiments were undertaken, each with from 30 to 50 college students as subjects. Each involved a sequence of three practice problems without feedback followed by a criterion problem. The problems involved a matrix of numbers to be added. The investigators found that when the practice problems and the criterion problems were structurally similar, those subjects who had had problem-solving experience tended to find shortcuts that helped them find a solution more often than did those subjects not having had problem-solving experience. However, when the practice problems and criterion problems differed considerably, those subjects having had experience tended to search for a shortcut unsuccessfully and thus required a longer time to find the solution than those subjects not having problem experiences.

The above study emphasizes the need for teachers to provide purposeful clarification of the goals of instruction and to be aware of the impact that the introduction to a given topic will have on future learnings.

SET AND CREATIVITY

Kramer, Tegan, and Knauber (1970) assessed the effect of informational pre-sets on baccalaureate nursing students. Their study focused on the creative use of library resources by students. "Creative" was defined as an uncommon or novel response reported to be workable. Their investigation was a replication of Hyman's (1964) study in which it was demonstrated that informational pre-sets affect the solving of a given task and enhance or hinder the formation of creative or uncommon solutions.

A bibliography was considered to be a limiting type of "advance organizer" or pre-set, because it structures material to be learned according to topics and prominent authors. Students were given the explanation that, in order to allow freedom of choice, a bibliography would not be given for the child area of nursing. Four experimental groups were presented with both common and uncommon ways of obtaining information. For example, reading a pediatrics textbook and using the bibliography at the end of each chapter, if additional source material was needed, was deemed common. In contrast, forming an informational reading and discussion group in which other students would report and critique what they had read was considered uncommon. Critical pre-sets were given to two of the experimental groups. One group was asked to list the disadvantages of the common solutions; the other was asked to list the disadvantages of the uncommon solutions. The remaining two experimental groups were given constructive pre-sets: one group was asked to list the advantages of the common solutions; the other was asked to list the advantages of the uncommon solutions. A control group of students was given no pre-set but was asked to list all solutions considered to be effective, as well as stating the advantages and disadvantages of each. Six weeks later all students were asked to list the solutions they had *actually used* in obtaining information.

It was found that there were significant differences in the occurrence of the uncommon responses in the group receiving the pre-set of being asked to list the disadvantages of common solutions. This group came up with many more unusual responses than the other three experimental groups but not significantly more than the control group, which had no informational input in terms of suggested solutions at all. This led the investigators to suggest that the general information given to *all* students—that of freedom to select material for themselves—was *in fact* a pre-set in itself.

This study lends support to the notion that teachers do affect student creative problem-solving behavior through the use of specific sets or directions. It further indicated that specific pre-sets tend to lose their power over time. The results suggest that specific pre-sets can transfer to other common or uncommon solutions to problems. It is interesting to note that the students stated far more unusual solutions than the faculty had anticipated!

SUMMARY

Preinstructional set can vary in length and elaborateness. Its purpose is to clarify the goals of instruction, motivate students to learn, and help students to see the relevance of the learning task. Set assists in organizing information by providing a common frame of reference. Set gives students an attitude of mind that helps them to accept or reject learning experiences. Because learning is a sequential process in which past learning forms the foundation for future learning, set helps students toward a cognitive bridge from one topic to another.

7

Achieving Closure

Closure is achieved when the major purposes and principles of a class, a course, or a program have been completed. Closure is complementary to set induction. It links the new knowledge to past knowledge and acts as a cognitive link to future learnings. Closure is of importance before going on to a new topic. It should provide more than a summary or review of what has been said.

EFFECT OF CLOSURE

Johnson (1965) draws a distinction between instructional closure and cognitive closure. He differentiates between the two by stating that instructional closure is reached when the class is completed and the *teacher* has shown the link between past knowledge and new knowledge. On the other hand, cognitive closure is reached when the *student* has reached closure and made the association between the old and new learnings. It can readily be seen that it is the latter—cognitive closure—that provides the more relevant learning goal.

The concept of organization and meaning in learning can be described in the principle as stated by Blair (1948): learning proceeds more rapidly and is retained longer when that which is learned possesses meaning, organization, and structure. After all, the major purpose for education is that it should serve us in the future. Transfer cannot occur by itself. It needs to be fostered by teaching behaviors. Closure is one teaching behavior that can assist the student in drawing meaningful relationships and forming an organization for transfer.

In testing the effects of cognitive closure on the achievement of ninth grade students, a study by Johnson (1965) indicated that cognitive closure as perceived by the student was positively associated with both immediate and delayed performance on tests of achievement. His findings give further support to the notion that learner achievement is significantly affected by the way in which the learner perceives the learning set as well as whether or not the set is perceived to be fulfilled by the student. In brief, both perceived learner set and perceived cognitive closure affect learner achievement. In addition to content achievement, it was found that students with perceived cognitive closure participated with greater willingness in subsequent learning experiences.

HELPING STUDENTS TOWARD CLOSURE

Allen and Ryan (1969) suggest three useful approaches to assist students toward closure, as well as to help the teacher ascertain whether closure has been achieved. These are:

1. *Review and summary*
   During a discussion with students, many different situations can be described, and students may respond in a variety of ways to the topic under discussion. While exploring a topic, it is not unusual for students to stray from the topic to tangential points or unfruitful paths. In order to give meaning, thrust, and organization to a free discussion, it is necessary for the teacher to listen to the meaning of what is being said, inventory comments, and abstract the ideas in order to summarize succinctly and help give the students a capsule summary of the salient points made by the group.

2. *Application of what has been learned to similar examples*
   Comparing the summarized ideas with a model of the structure of the content under consideration assists students in organizing the new information. For example, if students were discussing the care of immobile patients, a general discussion of the specific problems presented by each of the student's patients would bring forth much data. The teacher might, then, compare the summarized problems of these patients to a model of the problems of immobilization as generalized from groups of patients. By reinforcing the main points brought out

by the students, and tying these points to previous learnings, the teacher can assist the students to extract generalizations from the specific aspects of the topic.

3. *Extend what has been learned to new situations*
   This teaching behavior helps students toward transfer of knowledge from one situation to another. For example, following a discussion emphasizing the need to protect patients with debilitating conditions from external infections, asking students about other situations in which patients should be especially protected will help them to gain understanding that any patient with suppressed immunity factors is particularly susceptible to infection.

CLOSURE AND FEELING OF ACHIEVEMENT

In addition to pulling together the major points and acting as a cognitive link between past knowledge and new knowledge, closure provides students with a needed feeling of achievement. By providing closure the teacher can use students' contributions and fit them into a meaningful whole in order to help students to incorporate new ideas into their cognitive structure. Everyone has had the experience of being involved in a group that seemingly has failed in its decision-making process. The skillful leader who can order all the comments, point out areas of agreement and disagreement, and help the group toward defining next steps is achieving closure.

CLOSURE AND TRANSFER OF LEARNING

As previously stated, in addition to providing a sense of accomplishment, closure should provide value for the student. Transfer is perhaps the most significant criterion of learning. It refers to the extent to which knowledge and abilities learned in one situation will apply to a new and different situation. There are two major principles pertaining to transfer that are relevant to closure. The first is that transfer occurs when there is a recognized similarity between the learning situation and the transfer situation. The key word here is *recognized*, which implies that it is recognized by the learner. By pointing out other situations in which the generalizations under consideration will apply, transfer is being reinforced. This principle has been supported by experimental evidence (Humphreys, 1951), and the theory underlying transfer is that learning experiences with "identical elements" help students to generalize to new situations.

The second general principle of transfer applicable to closure is that transfer will occur to the extent that students expect it to occur (Saupe, 1961). Here it is not sufficient for new situations to have identical elements only with the learning ones or for students to know generalizations. In addition, students must perceive the identical elements in the new situation or recognize that the generalizations apply to the new situation. The study of organizational theory may lead to an understanding of the way complex organizations are structured, but it will not necessarily help a nursing student to understand the hospital as a complex organization unless the knowledge is applied to several types of organizations with the expectation that such knowledge is both usable and will assist the learner in the future.

USE OF CLOSURE

Closure is an appropriate activity to perform before going on to any new concept, idea, or problem. Because it is complementary to set induction, closure can be combined with establishing set. There are times, however, when closure is particularly relevant, such as at the end of a class session. Teachers often do not allow sufficient time for closure. Rather, they wait until the last minute of the class and become aware of the time because students are shuffling in their seats and the classroom door is being opened by the next group of students. With this interference, the closure may consist of a hurried one sentence summary followed by "That's it for today" with students scarcely listening at all.

The opposite can also occur. The students may achieve closure before the teacher! In this case, the teacher is dragging out points that are obvious and is taking a longer time to summarize than it took the group to bring forth the ideas in the first place. Under these circumstances, the teacher is belaboring the point in an unfruitful way. When a class is finished, it is finished; attempting to keep students to the appointed hour will only mean that they are physically present.

Closure is suitable for the completion of a unit of study or a course. Ways of achieving closure might include a case study; reading a poem that draws together the ideas to be conveyed; or presenting an analogy or short story that is read or distributed. The major idea that the instructor wishes to leave with the student can frequently be dramatically illustrated.

SUMMARY

Closure, as a teaching technique, helps students to abstract the very major ideas presented in a class, a teaching unit, or a course. It provides a link between what has been learned to the application of the knowledge. Closure is important because organization and meaningful learning assist in transfer in forming relationships. Furthermore, closure helps to give students a feeling of accomplishment and satisfaction in what they have learned.

PART 2

STRATEGIES FOR TEACHING GROUPS OF STUDENTS

8

Teaching by Lecture

The lecture is perhaps the oldest teaching strategy for large group teaching. Long before the invention of the printing press, groups of scholars sat with their tutor, listened, and took notes on his wise words. Because books remained expensive for some time following the invention of printing, the only way that a person could become educated was by the transmission of information through the teacher. As textbooks became more readily available, the lecture in the college and university was employed to reinforce and supplement written reference materials. Suffice it to say that the lecture should never be used for reading aloud from the textbook!

A deductive strategy is most commonly used in teaching by lecture. The teacher begins with a definition of the concepts or principles, illustrates them with examples, unfolds their implications, and provides closure by helping the students incorporate the new ideas into their schemes of cognitive structure. This type of teaching provides immediate reinforcement of the rule or principle being discussed. Presenting rules first can be effective because it can be more useful to the nursing student to remember a general statement; for example, that an increase in tissue or fluid in the cranium will lead to increased intracranial pressure rather than remembering that a cerebral vascular accident, a tumor, or trauma will all lead to increased intracranial pressure.

CAUTIONS IN THE USE OF FORMAL LECTURE

A formal lecture is one in which the lecturer does all of the talking. It is organized for the participants, and decisions are made in advance of the presentation. The disadvantages to this type of teaching strategy are that the "telling" technique is often an indication of subject matter domination in the learning process. Too much emphasis is put on certain facts and materials to be learned and too little on the learning process itself, and on the desired results. In this way it may encourage the retention of facts as an end in itself. Furthermore, exposition as an approach to teaching tends to emphasize the wants and desires of the lecturer to the exclusion of the students' needs. It fosters dependence on the teacher as the final authority, thus inhibiting the exploratory aspect of learning. Most important, the formal lecture creates a passive type of learning that tends not to be retained. In the words of Gayles (1966),

> The lecture at its worst consists of transferring the notes of the teacher to the notebooks of the students without passing through the minds of either.

The lecture as a teaching method is being denounced mostly as a reaction against its long years of misuse and overuse. Its misuse occurs when it is used when other strategies would achieve the particular learning objectives, as active learning is preferable to passive learning. College students often state that they enjoy lectures, but it should be borne in mind that when the instructor capsulizes all the pertinent information, students are saved a trip to the library to dig it out for themselves. Every problem solved by the teacher is one less problem for the student to solve. Attitudes, skills, and feelings cannot be learned through pure "show and tell" procedures.

Kaufmann (1977) issues a scathing statement about lectures in higher education. He states that most are a waste of time and points out that if the lecturer does not write a lecture out, chances are that it will be greatly inferior to something available in print that could be assigned to students to read instead. And, he goes on to say, if the lecturer does write the lecture out, there seems to be no need to read it because it could be made available to the students to read for themselves!

There are, of course, reasons that lectures are not uniformly excellent in higher education. Satterfield (1978) estimates that the average lecturer speaks at the rate of 150 words per minute. This means that a 50-minute lecture produces 7,500 words! He also points out that very few writers could be as prolific, and at the same time exercise all the careful revisions required to produce an excellent treatise, using the number of words that lecturers must use during a given course that employs the lecture as the only teaching method. In view of all of the criticisms lodged against the college lecture, Satterfield (1978) summarizes the situation with a resigned statement. He points out that lecturing is likely to remain the most prevalent practice of college teaching. If this is so, and we have no reason to challenge his statement based on our own observations of teaching in schools of nursing, it behooves those who lecture to learn to do it with a moderate (at least) degree of skill.

ADVANTAGES OF THE LECTURE

In spite of the criticisms of the lecture method of teaching, there obviously must be many advantages to it, or this widespread teaching technique would not have survived for so many generations of college students. The specific advantages of the lecture method of teaching include:

1. It can help to emphasize and clarify important points and thus channel the thinking of a group of students in the given direction.
2. The lecture can enliven facts and ideas that might seem tedious on the pages of a book.
3. Lectures can expose large groups of students to authorities in order to share first-hand experiences. It is indeed inspirational for students to experience the enthusiasm and excitement that a nursing leader feels for our profession. This excitement can be transmitted to large numbers of students when such a person is invited to speak to and with students on campus. A nurse returning from another country can share perceptions of a different culture, as well as add a fresh way of viewing nursing problems in our nation, with groups of students by lecture.
4. An individual who is testing a nursing theory can share ideas before publication and thus give students the advantage of hearing truly original ideas.
5. The teacher's experience, enthusiasm, and special way of organizing materials, presented with masterful delivery, can serve as a motivation and inspiring experience for students. For introducing a new topic or concept, explaining a process, telling how something is done, giving perspective to the work of the class, or summarizing what has been learned, the lecture has no equal.

LECTURE-DISCUSSION

The informal lecture, or lecture-discussion as it is frequently called, is perhaps the most common teaching strategy used in classroom teaching in colleges. With this method the presentation is supplemented by audiovisual aids, and students are encouraged to interrupt for questions, comments, and clarification.

McKeachie (1963) states that the use of both, lectures and discussions, is a logical and popular choice in courses in which the instructors wish not only to give information but also to develop concepts. The lecture can effectively present new research findings; the discussion can give students opportunities to analyze the studies, find relationships, and develop generalizations. By participating actively in discussion, students not only learn the generalization but also develop skill in critical thinking as well.

As with all teaching strategies, it is imperative that the teacher have a clear-cut purpose for what is to be accomplished. In organizing a class around a lecture and lecture-discussion method, the teacher plans the class so that it will progress in an orderly manner. A short overview helps students to focus on the topic; a creative way of producing set helps students to enter into the class both cognitively and affectively. The teacher plans for the supporting data needed to substantiate views and has additional material ready if further clarification is necessary. However, merely because the teacher has the examples does not constitute rationale for using all of them. Repetition beyond that needed to assure understanding tends to be boring.

ORGANIZING THE LECTURE

Foley and Smilansky (1980) offer some excellent advice for organizing a lecture. Essentially, a lecture should be organized into three parts: an introduction, body, and conclusion. It adheres to the old teaching adage of "tell them what you are going to tell them, tell them; and then tell them what you told them."

The Introduction

The component of set induction in Chapter 6 applies to the introduction of a lecture. All too often lecturers begin by merely stating the topic (e.g., "Today we will discuss the care of the patient who is anxious") and then proceed immediately to the body of the lecture. An effective introduction to a lecture delineates the specific topics that will be covered and states the order in which they will be discussed. In introducing the topic of caring for patients who are anxious the lecturer could say: "Today we are going to discuss anxiety and the ways in which your patients may manifest it. We will define anxiety, discuss its prevalence, its origins in terms of psychoanalytic and other theories, the precipitating factors, and the major ways in which anxiety can be alleviated." Sometimes opening a lecture with a series of questions may peak the interest of students.

In order to assist students in following the organization of the lecture, an outline is helpful. This can be written on a chalkboard or shown on an overhead projector. The entire outline can be presented at once to allow students to view the total lecture organization before its beginning, or the teacher may wish to vary this by presenting points one by one and adding to the outline as each new idea is presented. For the latter plan, an overhead projector provides an excellent means for adding points, while allowing students to keep the preceding ones in view. Either using overlays to build up the outline, or covering up on the transparency the ideas yet to be discussed using a piece of opaque paper, can be effective. Such an outline helps the teacher follow with the planned sequence, as well as allowing students to contribute in a focused manner. It assists the teacher in avoiding unnecessary repetition or gaps in presentation.

The ground rules for the lecture should be stated. For example, the lecturer may not wish to interrupt the presentation with questions from students. In that case, it is important to state that a specified period of time at the conclusion of the lecture will be reserved for questions. Or the lecturer may prefer to have students ask questions at the conclusion of each segment of the lecture. In either case, it is essential that the lecturer repeat the student's questions so that all in the room have heard the question before the lecturer launches into the answer or discussion.

Body of Lecture

The body of the lecture should be organized so that information flows logically from one point to another. It should not deviate from the boundaries established in the introduction. Poor planning, or to be more precise, inadequate planning, results in rambling presentations and frequent digressions that make it difficult for the audience to pay attention to what is being said. Some lecturers are overly enthusiastic in their approach and attempt to include too much material in the lecture. As a matter of fact, too much material is frequently the result of inadequate preparation. It takes longer to prepare carefully for a short lecture (or a short article) than to allow oneself the luxury of going on and on.

During a lecture, the teacher should be sensitive to feedback from the students, particularly the nonverbal cues that can indicate lack of understanding, boredom, or daydreaming. It is important to emphasize that although such cues as yawning, whispering, or sleeping may indicate that the material or its presentation is not stimulating to students, the teacher should take into account other reasons, such as poor ventilation, inadequate lighting, or the time of the day, as other possible causes of inattentive behavior from students. A droning voice on a warm summer day following lunch does lull students to sleep! Note how an information-giving television program, such as a news commentary, is paced. Short bits of information are given, interspersed with a videotaped "on the scene" report, still pictures, or illustrations of the event. Remember the reason Hayden suddenly raised the volume on his *Surprise Symphony*. It was to awaken the slumberers during a chamber music concert! Varying the stimuli by these means and such others as shifting from expository teaching to discussion become essential to maintain or regain the active involvement of the learner.

Eye contact with the audience is also important. Beginning, or insecure, lecturers sometimes keep their eyes glued to the back of the room instead of scanning the entire group. Moving about provides a changing focus for the audience and varies the stimuli. However, too much moving can be distracting. There really are no hard and fast rules for improving presentation styles, because each person has a unique personality and should develop his or her own style. Summaries of research on teaching effectiveness consistently cite qualities such as warmth, enthusiasm, and motivation as features of the effective lecturer and instructor (Foley & Smilansky, 1980). How does one demonstrate these elusive characteristics? Unfortunately, no magic formula exists. It has been suggested that one ask for help from colleagues who can give specific and constructive feedback after attending a lecture. Videotaping a lecture and reviewing the tape repeatedly has helped many novice (or experienced) lecturers to improve their presentation styles.

The Conclusion

The principles discussed in Chapter 7 on achieving closure relate to this part of the lecture. All too often lecturers simply run out of time and hastily conclude what they want to say. The salient points should be repeated, and if the lecture will continue on the same topic or one closely related, the content of the summary can provide the bridge to the next lecture. Sometimes questions are effective. For example, in discussing the concept *anxiety* students could be asked to identify symptoms of anxiety in each patient they care for during their next clinical experience.

AUDIOVISUAL AIDS

It has been pointed out by Bugelski (1964) that the educational world has been slow to take advantage of technological advances that can make teaching more effective. Several reasons for this reluctance have been offered. One is the "cultural lag" of simply not being aware of the new aids for teaching. Other reasons include vague fears that the machines will take over the teacher's functions, rather than viewing these aids as adjuncts to the teaching process. In order not to limit communication with students to voice and gesture alone, other audiovisual aids should be used.

Teachers have been using illustrations as long as they have been teaching. Such great teachers as Socrates and Archimedes drew pictures and diagrams in the sand to illustrate their points. Because it is thought we remember only 10 percent of what we hear and 20 percent of what we see, retention is increased by using illustrations. The chalkboard is one of the oldest and most used of audiovisual aids. It needs no explanation, except to point out that its use for drawing illustrations greatly enhances the clarity of some materials. For some inexplicable reason, when teachers draw on the board they usually feel compelled to apologize for their lack of artistic ability before or immediately following completion of their masterpiece. In addition to drawing attention to the very aspect they wish to avoid, this remark can become somewhat disconcerting to students who hear the same apology from teacher after teacher. Remember that no student expects a nursing teacher to be a van Gogh or a medical illustrator. Nursing instructors who are unduly sensitive about their lack of artistry might wish to carefully draw their pictures on the board before class. One effective use of the chalkboard involves drawing on the board, erasing the board leaving the outline (not discernible to the class) and whipping up the picture by tracing the outline in front of the class! Another idea is to use the artistic skills of students. In addition to receiving a clear illustration, this can serve as a way to recognize special talents of students.

The advantages of using colored chalk in illustrating a lecture are dramatically told by Eleanor Clark, the 1981 Council for Advancement and Support of Education's "Professor of the Year" (Ingalls, 1981). She states that slides, overhead transparencies, and material presented by means of opaque projectors all present students with a whole picture, whereas drawing on the chalkboard allows the students' minds to follow what the teacher is doing rather than wandering to other topics.

Overhead Projector

The overhead projector is perhaps the easiest of all of the audiovisual aids to use. This optical instrument enlarges a 10-inch transparency to viewing size on a projection screen within a distance of a few feet. Because it is operated from the front of the class, the teacher controls the management rather than relying on a technical aid. The teacher thus avoids distracting instructions and can integrate the material from the transparency with the presentation naturally and without losing eye contact with the class. The transparency can be a diagram or written or pictorial illustration. Reed (1968) lists several pertinent points for the teacher to observe when operating the overhead projector in order to increase the effectiveness of the material presented. The placement of the projector and screen in relation to the class is of importance. Both the teacher and the head of the projector can obstruct the view of material for the student unless the screen is carefully placed. If the head of the projector is not placed at a right angle to the screen, distortion of the image, known as "keystoning," will occur. This creates an image larger at the top than bottom. To gain better visibility in the classroom, placing the screen higher and slanting the screen will prevent the "keystone" effect. Because the light of the overhead projector tends to draw students' eyes to it, it should be turned off when not specifically in use. Also, while changing the transparencies, the light should be turned off to avoid the phenomenon of visual confusion.

Transparencies for the overhead projector can be easily made by the instructor by writing with a waxed pencil or special felt-tipped pen. Duplicating illustrations or prepared materials can be done by using a specially treated transparency and a thermal duplicator. The materials are either color sensitive or color can be added by special overlay material or colored pens or pencils. It takes but a few moments to make an attractive transparency. The most dramatic transparency illustrates a single thought or comparison. Too much detail in a transparency can confuse viewers and lessen the impact of the visual image as a communications tool. A good transparency contains one idea, visual identification, legible writing (at least ¼" high), and imaginative design. Color should be used for emphasis of a particular part of the transparency. Overuse of color will detract from its value. Commercially prepared transparencies are available for purchase from textbook companies. These transparencies are prepared in color with overlays, which assist in giving added dimension to the material. In addition to the anatomical charts, to which this material readily lends itself, nursing examples include such lessons as preparing and calculating solutions, the patient and circulatory disorders, and the patient and fluid balance.

The addition of an attachment, which polarizes light on specially treated overlay materials or materials laminated onto the transparency, gives the effect of movement. This is particularly effective when motion adds to the learning experience, as with the circulatory system. It also serves as a stimulus variation.

Slides and Film Strips

Slides that are well produced provide the clearest and most accurate images of all audiovisual aids. They can be changed with ease, and modern classrooms include equipment that enables the lecturer to control the pace at which the slides are changed. The lecturer does not have to lose eye contact with the audience, and slides can be easily integrated into the lecture with a minimum of distraction to the audience.

Foley and Smilansky (1980) offer four points for use with instructional media that are particularly applicable to the use of slides. First, they should be carefully incorporated into the verbal presentation, with the objective of illustrating and clarifying particular ideas, rather than provide a major focus. Second, media should only be used when they enhance understanding of the subject matter. Third, audiovisual aids should be clearly visible and audible. Too much information on a slide detracts rather than clarifies. Finally, preview all of the slides before presentation to be certain that they are in order, right side up, and that the screen can be lowered at the appropriate time.

Slides and film strips are commonly used to illustrate a real-life situation. For example, in helping nursing students to describe the appearance of a patient, color slides of patients who are cyanotic, or who have skin rashes, could be used as illustrations. Commercially prepared film strips illustrate basic nursing procedures.

MOTION PICTURES AND TELEVISION

When sound and motion are added to pictures, their usefulness as a teaching aid is multiplied by both learning retention and transfer, because more senses are brought into play by the student. Both motion pictures and television are very useful tools for the teaching-learning process.

Motion pictures and television can be employed as media to present more complex and lifelike stimuli in the classroom. By means of closed-circuit television or videotape, clinical situations can be brought to the classroom for discussion and critique. Time-lapsed videotapes can tele-scope time and permit students to understand the problems of chronic disabilities and their effects on patients, for example, without waiting the several years for the process to unfold. Edited tapes provide teachers with a tool that can specifically suit their own purposes. Commercially produced motion pictures provide the teacher with the advantage of having a readymade teaching aid. In some locales, schools of nursing are pooling their faculty resources by videotaping expert lectures and thus bringing master teachers to other schools of nursing when it fits into the borrower's course plan. This plan could be offered, either through vid-eotape recordings or educational broadcast television to bring nursing's leaders to every school of nursing in much the same way as, several decades ago, Dr. Harvey White and seven Nobel prize winners and other distinguished scientists brought an excellent basic college physics course to many universities—an array of talent virtually impossible for any one university to gather for itself.

Unfortunately, the progress of television on college campuses has been slow. Eurich (1964) attributes this to the fear of college professors that they will somehow become obsolete. He points out that the same objection was made at Oxford and Cambridge universities at the end of the nineteenth century when the "university lecture" was added to sup-plement the tutorial method of instruction. What actually happened at those two universities was that when relieved of the responsibility of preparing for lectures, faculty members could devote themselves to guiding student progress, individually and in small groups. The student benefited from the opportunity to hear the very best lecturers in each field.

In a study designed to compare student achievement and attitudes under three conditions: off-campus television instruction, on-campus television instruction, and instructor-present, no television instruction, Dreher and Beatty (1958) found few significant differences in achieve-ment for any of the conditions or subject matters. The subjects taught were psychology, economics, basic communications, and creative arts. Students with low grade-point averages did significantly better with tele-vised instruction in both psychology and economics. The off-campus television students tended to favor television instruction, while the on-campus television group tended to be more disapproving than off-campus students. The nontelevision, instructor-present group tended to be least critical of their courses of all. It is, of course, important to add that the variables included more than television or lack of it. Those faculty who prepared classes for the television presentations had at their disposal innumerable resources, including graphic arts specialists, technical advisors, and colleagues. Seldom does an individual college teacher have such resources. Therefore, because television teaching is more public in both resources and critique, it helps the teacher to present material in varying ways, which in themselves lead to more effective teaching. In addition, the newness and convenience of taking a course in the comfort of one's own home tends to influence students. This "Hawthorne Effect" presents a very real problem for global studies of educational methodology research, and for this reason results of such studies must be viewed with caution. Unfortunately, relatively few studies have been undertaken for a period longer than one semester. McKeachie (1963) suggests that television may be particularly valuable for those courses involving demonstrations.

All of the aforementioned teaching aids require some degree of hardware. Every teacher has had the disconcerting experience of having difficulty with the equipment or having a film arrive too late to be of use in planned learning sequence. Although most of the newer equipment is easier and handier to use, it is important to advise that the machines should be tried out before class. Films or videotapes that are difficult to see or hear detract from the learning situation. Problems can and do occur.

Although it is perfectly true that varying the stimuli within a class period is necessary in order to increase the attention span and receptivity of students, random selection of materials for the sake of the use of hardware alone leads to unproductive results. Audiovisual materials should not be used for their own sake but rather for their ability to communicate more fully to students.

RESEARCH ON TEACHING BY LECTURE

The research studies focusing on teaching by lecture compare it with teaching by group discussion. The results are largely inconclusive, very possibly because of the lack of differentiation of the desired outcomes. When one asks whether lecture is better than discussion, the appropriate counter is "For what goals?" When the effectiveness of a lecture-demonstration technique was compared with that of a problem-solving discussion in a college science course, the lecture-demonstration method proved superior when the criterion test was a test of specific knowledge. However, when the criterion test was a problem-solving and scientific attitude measurement, then the discussion technique was superior (Barnard, 1942). These findings have been supported by other studies (Dawson, 1956; DiVesta, 1954).

Considerable research has focused on the size of the lecture audience. Is a small class more effective in terms of learning outcomes than a large one? As with much research in education, there has been a lack of conclusive experimental support for either position. Most teachers believe small classes are superior to large ones. McKeachie (1963) sums up the class size dilemma by saying that large lecture classes are not generally inferior to smaller lecture classes when the traditional tests of achievement are used as a criterion. If the role of the instructor as an information giver is stressed, then information-giving is a one-way process, and the size of the group is not a relevant variable. In fact, the size of the group need be limited only to being audible. It has been suggested, in fact, that in expository teaching the size of the group may be a motivational factor in teacher preparation and planning for the lecture. However, when other objectives are measured, such as problem solving, student interaction, and so forth, the larger classes are less effective. Furthermore, both students and faculty feel that teaching is more effective in smaller classes. Regardless of whether there is validity in these findings, movement toward larger classes usually meets with resistance from both groups.

McKeachie (1963) summarizes the role of the lecture in higher education by pointing out that research results provide little basis for a supportable answer. The research results do not contradict, and sometimes support, the notion that the lecture is an effective way of communicating information. However, there is evidence that other methods of teaching may be more effective than expository techniques when achieving higher cognitive and attitudinal objectives.

SUMMARY

Although teaching by lecture is a traditional and widespread teaching practice in institutions of higher learning, there has been remarkably little investigation about its effectiveness. Ausubel (1963, p. 19) defends it by saying:

The art and science of presenting ideas and information meaningfully and effectively—so that clear, stable, and unambiguous meanings emerge and are retained over a long period of time as an organized body of knowledge—is really the principal function of pedagogy. . . . The job of selecting, organizing, presenting, and translating subject-matter content in a developmentally appropriate manner . . . is the work of a master teacher and is hardly a task to be disdained.

Many teachers favor lecturing because it is efficient and takes less time than helping students to discover principles for themselves. Lecturing gives the teacher control over the learning process. It assists in giving students an organized view of nursing as a discipline because the experienced nurse who teaches is a more effective organizer of nursing than the novice nursing student.

A major disadvantage of teaching by lecture is that although the students acquire information in the form of facts and generalizations, they frequently do not have the opportunity to manipulate the generalizations for themselves. Students may not have the opportunity to find the information in their own cognitive storage systems when needed to solve problems for themselves.

9

Teaching by Seminar

Anytime more than two persons gather together to discuss an idea, debate a point, analyze an issue, or work together to gain consensus, it becomes a group discussion. Discussion may be defined as the free and unhampered consideration of a problem by a cooperative group of persons talking together under the guidance of one of its members (Keltner, 1956).

The small group discussion allows students to interact with one another and with their instructor, to give as well as take, and to develop confidence in their own ideas and their abilities to express themselves with clarity and logic. Discussions bring about divergent views and help students toward a more creative approach to problem solving.

Small group instruction can be employed in several ways in the nursing school curriculum. Patterned after a common procedure in universities, large classes may be sectioned to allow students adequate opportunity for discussion. A large number of students may have been presented with the same ideas through expository teaching. Because of the size of the class, interaction between students and between student and teacher is limited. Following immediately, or later during the week, students in smaller groups meet with their own section instructor to exchange ideas. The instructor, in order to perform a consultant role, would need to have firsthand knowledge of the expository session. Students are provided the opportunity to raise questions about points not clear to them and test their own thoughts.

Group conferences, following clinical experiences, provide the opportunities for group problem solving and comparing and contrasting patients' nursing problems. It is in the postclinical nursing conference that a great deal of discovery or inductive teaching-learning can take place. For example, if the nursing problem under discussion is nursing interventions in caring for patients with long-term disabilities, the students may have cared for patients with such problems as sensory deprivation, locomotor difficulties, or chronic pulmonary problems. In addition to the subject-matter sampling that can take place in this way, students also may seek assistance from peers to help them identify alternative ways of solving nursing care problems. In addition to the one patient each student may have cared for, vicarious experiences are multiplied by the number of students in the group.

SEMINAR TEACHING

Not all small groups can be considered seminars. It is a misuse of the term when it is used to indicate a course with small enrollment, or an undirected, unfocused discussion by instructor or students or both. Guinée (1966) defines the seminar as a form of class organization that uses a scientific approach to the analysis of a problem chosen for discussion. The seminar is guided discussion with the student taking the intellectual initiative. The teacher is a member of the group, sometimes acting as leader, other times as consultant. Discussion involves the sharing of ideas and information, the give and take of opinions and exploration of problems and questions.

Discussion assumes that desirable learning outcomes are possible when students can argue, judge data, draw conclusions, compare, and contrast. The group experiences center on the learning activity rather than the teacher or subject matter as determined by the teacher. The value of discussion is in its provision for student involvement and the practice it affords students in assessing, relating, summarizing, and applying ideas. Discussion techniques can promote deeper understanding of learnings as well as affect attitudes, interests, and develop desirable interpersonal relationships.

RESEARCH ON SEMINAR LEARNING

The research pertaining to student-centered versus instructor-centered teaching is relevant to seminar teaching and learning. A wide variety of teaching methods are described by such labels as "student-centered," "nondirective," "group-centered," or "democratic" discussions. All these techniques have in common the breaking away from the traditional instructor dominated classroom in order to encourage greater student responsibility and participation.

As we discussed previously, a major reason that it is difficult to gather evidence about the superiority of one teaching method over another is because it is difficult to delineate the teaching method that is most productive when one deals with "learning" in global terms. Moreover, the standard of measure for most studies on teaching methods in higher education is the traditional achievement test of knowledge acquisition rather than tests of application or problem-solving skills.

Although scores on objective examinations are little affected by teaching method (McKeachie, 1966), other factors indicate that student behavior apart the usual testing situation may be influenced in the direction of educational goals by student-centered teaching.

One study (Lyle, 1958) compared a problem-oriented approach to the conventional lecture-discussion-text procedures. The conventional group was found to be superior to the problem-oriented approach in achievement. However, when students were asked to submit a question for the final examination, more students in the conventional groups wrote factual-type questions than did those in the problem-centered group. The problem-centered group submitted more "thought" questions.

Gibb and Gibb (1952) report that students taught by active-participation methods are significantly more accomplished than students taught by the traditional lecture-discussion methods in role flexibility and insight. They also found that these same students were rated by peers in nonclassroom situations as high in leadership, popularity, and group membership skills.

McKeachie (1966) summarizes the results of research on student-centered teaching methods as not impressive, but supporting of the theory that student-centered methods are effective in achieving higher-order cognitive objectives and in producing noncognitive changes.

ADVANTAGES OF SEMINAR LEARNING

An understanding of the group process is an important objective of the school of nursing curriculum. Nurses, as well as other health professionals, work together in every aspect of the helping endeavor. We work as team leaders and team members in providing direct patient care services; we collaborate with other health professionals in the planning of health care; we work with patients and their families; and we serve as members of committees, boards, and commissions both in the community and in our educational institutions. The seminar method of teaching provides first-hand experience in group decision making and group problem solving.

An important contribution of the group problem-solving process is the effect it has in modifying an individual's own style of solving problems through exposure to how others solve problems. Individual solutions are built one upon the other, thus giving the student many more alternative solutions than might have been possible previously.

The usual process followed in group problem solving is that group members exchange information relevant to the problem, one or more solutions based on the information are proposed, and, finally, agreement is reached. In the early phase, that of exchanging information relevant to the problem, students have the opportunity to review knowledge pertaining to the problem. Resources, such as reference materials and consultants, can be brought in or sought by the group.

VARIABLES IN GROUP PRODUCTIVITY AND GROUP SATISFACTION

There is a rich body of research on small groups. We will limit our discussions in this chapter to groups formed for the purpose of meeting educational objectives—task-oriented groups. It must be noted that students may or may not select the group they are in, or may or may not have the option of attending group meetings. In schools of nursing where students progress together throughout their nursing school experiences, a small group of classmates may well take on the characteristics of what Cooley (1909) terms the "primary group." These characteristics include a strong sense of individual identity to the group. It involves a great feeling of sympathy and mutual identification with other members of the group. Group members consistently use the word "we" when referring to their group. Such groups cannot tolerate antagonism because the primary relationship entails a positive valuing of one another, a sense of "we-ness," of belonging together and sharing a common identity (Broom & Selznick, 1958). An example of such primary group behavior is demonstrated when a delegation of nursing students is selected to protest such action as one of their members failing a course.

Three of the most important variables pertaining to group productivity and group satisfaction are group leadership, group size, and the communication structure. We will consider each of these factors next.

Group Leadership

Much has been written about group leadership. Secord and Backman (1964) point out that many small groups have two different leadership needs. The first is a task leader who supplies ideas and guides the group toward problem solution. The other leadership need is what they term the social-emotional role to help boost group morale.

Some groups experience difficulty maintaining a balance between the task orientation and the social-emotional functions of the group. Bales and Slater (1955) explain the events leading to hostility toward a task-oriented leader. Initially the group members feel satisfied with the progress they are making toward the task. If the group leader utilizes prestige given to the leader to talk a large proportion of the time, eventually hostility will be aroused from some group members. They will eventually transfer some of their initially positive feelings toward the leader to another person who is less active but who expresses their own negative feelings. This latter person becomes the social-emotional leader in representing the values and attitudes that have been disturbed, deemphasized, threatened, or repressed by the task-oriented leader. It is when this occurs that true differentiation of the leadership role occurs.

Groups vary in the extent to which they emphasize task and social-emotional abilities as criteria for leadership. Bales and Slater (1955) suggest that the degree of role differentiation varies directly with the extent to which task functions are unrewarded or costly to group members. When a group experiences little satisfaction in working together toward a goal, the social-emotional functions and task functions tend to be centered on different persons. These conditions tend to occur in a group where there is lack of consensus on the goal, where communication skills are underdeveloped, and where there is little consensus on values and activities.

The implications for teachers indicate that any set of circumstances that reduces the need for differentiation of leadership roles will tend to keep the balance between the task accomplishment and the emotional needs of the group members. Thibaut and Kelley (1959) point out that hostility toward the leader and role differentiation are reduced when the leadership style encourages a wide distribution of directive acts so that no one person becomes the sole target of hostility. Thus, the democratic leader who encourages division of responsibility and participation in decisions may well be able to carry on both task and social-emotional roles.

An investigation conducted in a classroom situation indicates that arousal of hostility toward an instructor is a direct function of the extent to which the instructor violates the legitimate expectations of the students by following his or her own inclinations rather than the students' wishes (Horwitz, 1963). In this study, instructions were given in college ROTC classes too rapidly for the students to grasp them thoroughly. It was agreed that votes would be taken to determine if the instructions should be repeated before going on to the next task. In one group, called the teacher-centered condition, students were informed that the instructor's vote would have twice the weight of the students' combined vote. In the second group, called the student-centered condition, students were told that the instructor's vote would be weighted only one-fourth that of the student group. The actual votes were disregarded and the prearranged experimental conditions were substituted. It was announced to the teacher-centered group that the instructor favored going on to the next topic while slightly more than half of the students had voted to repeat the instructions. With these ratings it was legitimate to go on to another topic because the group had been told that extra weight would be given to the instructor's vote. When the same announcement was made to the student-centered group, the action was perceived as illegitimate because the instructor was arbitrarily reducing the weight given to the student's votes. Considerably more hostility toward the instructor was generated in the student-centered group.

Group Size

As anyone who has experienced the group process will attest, the larger a group becomes the less it is able to accomplish. Gibb (1951) suggests that idea productivity is a *negatively accelerated* increasing function of the size of a group. Much of this appears to be related to need satisfaction. If a group is very large, obviously the individual's needs cannot be met often, as each person must wait his or her turn. As is frequently observed, the rate of participation in small groups tends to be fairly equal among members, but in large groups the majority of the talking is done by the same few persons. Although the increase in size, theoretically, means that each individual will have the opportunity to learn from more persons, this advantage is counteracted by the factors just mentioned. Although the literature does not cite an optimum number for group productivity, many nursing schools vary the number of students for seminars between 10 and 20.

Communication Structure

The well-known phrase "let's sit in a circle" is frequently heard in teaching. Although many students complain that this seating arrangement is overdone, there is research evidence supporting this plan to facilitate communications. Individuals find it more satisfying to communicate directly with one another rather than receiving communications through a third party. This includes nonverbal communications as well as verbal. In fact, nonverbal communications depend on sight and, hence, are completely impossible if the individuals cannot view one another. Leavitt (1951) found that when he placed his subjects in a circle they communicated more freely with one another and expressed more need satisfaction. Face-to-face contact facilitates feedback.

ROLE OF INSTRUCTOR IN FACILITATING GROUP GOAL

Although the group leadership will change, depending on the objective of the group setting, the instructor is generally perceived as a leader by students because of the position. As such, it is the instructor's role to be knowledgeable in the subject under discussion in order to be a resource person. It is also the instructor's role to keep the group from floundering in an unproductive way. There are ways in which teachers can facilitate group discussions.

First, no matter what the objective of the small group discussion is, one common aspect is that it is the members of the group whose opinion, comments, or questions are being sought—not the teacher's. Speaking tends to be an occupational disease among college teachers. It takes much practice and soul-searching to reach the degree of teaching maturity that allows for patience with students and to not tell students either a solution or idea until they have had the opportunity to explore the issue thoroughly by themselves.

Because individuals tend to speak more when they know one another, instructors facilitate communications when encouraging a friendly environment, by helping students to know one another. In a large school it cannot be assumed that everyone knows one another. The introductory phase of the group process cannot be rushed or ignored. Experience teaches us that it generally takes several meetings.

Instructors can facilitate the group's goals by outlining what needs to be accomplished or the topic for discussion. They can do this themselves, or they can help the group do it for itself, depending on the objectives of the group meeting. This lends support to one of Hilgard's (1956, p. 486) learning theories—individuals need practice in setting realistic goals for themselves. If goals are set too low, little effort will be elicited; if too high, they may predetermine failure. Realistic goal setting leads to more satisfactory improvement than unrealistic goal setting.

In addition to knowing the structure of the subject to be discussed, instructors can help to create a climate for a free and unthreatening discussion. Knowing the students, instructors can draw out timid students by giving them opportunities to express themselves and reinforcing them for speaking. A somewhat shy student may not be able to discuss ideas simply because she or he is not aggressive enough to cut in on classmates' discussions. The teacher who is sensitive to nonverbal cues may facilitate this student's speaking by merely stating, "Mary, you look like you wish to add to this last statement." The instructor can help overeager students gain self-understanding of their need to be heard or dominate a conversation to the exclusion of others. The instructor, likewise, can assist the student who becomes unduly uneasy when verbally challenged. Faculty members often ask how one deals with the student who is aggressive, sensitive, or retiring. Because individuals differ so much, it is virtually impossible and extremely dangerous to suggest any approach without knowing all of the variables involved. Every approach to a student, as to a patient, is a hypothesis about human behavior. The sensitive instructor is alert to opportunities to try different approaches, seeks and accepts feedback, and attempts many alternatives to assist each student in the group.

CONDUCTING A DISCUSSION

Conducting a class discussion requires on-the-spot decisions, diagnoses, and formulating questions. In developing the skill of leading a class discussion, bear in mind that there is no such thing as a perfect discussion. However, some discussions are more effective than others in terms of student learnings and outcomes.

One of the first tasks the instructor must perform is to "get the ball rolling." When the teacher runs out of ideas, brainstorming is a technique that can get the group started thinking toward a solution to a problem. "Brainstorming" was first used in the business world. The rules of brainstorming are that group members give whatever idea occurs to them about a problem. Other members of the group are prohibited from evaluating the idea as presented but are encouraged to free associate and contribute their own ideas. De Cecco (1968) has summarized the studies made of the usefulness of this technique as follows: (1) training in brainstorming increases creative problem solving; (2) brainstorming produces more problem solutions than do methods that penalize bad ideas in some way; (3) more good ideas are produced with brainstorming than with conventional techniques; (4) extended efforts to produce ideas lead to an increased number of ideas and proportion of good ideas; and (5) students in creative problem-solving courses (which include brainstorming) obtain higher scores on tests of creative abilities than do students who have not had these courses. Although students do not evaluate ideas submitted immediately, there is a need to return later to determine the probable significance and worthiness of each idea. If not, it may turn out to be the kind of solution attributed to Will Rogers when he suggested that the best way to capture the enemy's submarines during the war was to heat the ocean to a sufficient degree to cause them to float to the surface. When asked how this could be accomplished, he replied "Don't bother me with the details. I'm an idea man!"

Once the group discussion is stated, there are ways to keep the discussion on the track. Taba (1967) suggests that there are four discussion leadership skills: focusing, refocusing, changing the focus, and recapping what has been said. Each will be discussed.

Focusing

People tend to indulge in associative thinking. They branch off from one idea to another. Providing that the group returns to the original task, associative thinking can be tolerated. But, unless brainstorming is the objective, it is the role of the discussion leader to ask a question that specifically sets the focus. Focusing questions may be open-ended, such as "Why do you think patients miss clinic appointments?", or they may be such that a single answer is appropriate to gather information.

Refocusing

Refocusing is necessary when the group has strayed from the original topic, and the discussion leader wishes the group to return to it. At times this is done directly such as saying "Let's go back to the topic at hand." It can be done more subtly when the teacher shifts the angle by repeating what a student has said and asks a question that prompts students back to the subject.

Changing the Focus

When a group has obviously discussed a topic sufficiently, and no new ideas or information are forthcoming, then it is usually time to change the focus. An example of this might be "Now that we have listed all the physiological changes occurring with advancing age we can think of, what other changes occur?"

Recapping

The recap is a brief version of a summary of what a group has said. Its purpose is to lift out ideas that have been offered in order to make them more understandable to the group and to set a clearer perspective. Recaps help students to see relationships and make conclusions.

DISCUSSION STOPPERS

Eaton, Davis, and Benner (1977) identified 11 teacher behaviors that inhibit student participation during discussions. They point to the necessity for teacher understanding of the reasons that classroom or conference discussions can fizzle out. They suggest that the teacher, often inadvertently, causes sluggish discussions that result in more teacher-talk than discussion from students. The 11 discussion stoppers they have identified are as follows:

1. *Insufficient "wait-time"*
   This occurs when teachers hasten to answer a question themselves, rephrase the question, or add further information to the question instead of allowing time for thoughtful responses from the students.
2. *The rapid reward*
   Rapid acceptance of a correct answer favors the faster thinker or speaker, whereas those in midthought are cut off prematurely. Although positive reinforcement is an important factor, too rapid or too forceful a reinforcement can prevent further extension of an idea by other students.

3. *The programmed answer*

   Examples within this group include questions that are really not questions and serve to irritate students and block further discussion. Eaton and her colleagues (1977) use the following question to illustrate this point, "Do you think it would be important to learn about different cultural patterns before doing community health nursing?" The teacher obviously has the answer in mind and is asking for students to confirm it. It is such an obvious question that few students would be willing to dignify it with a response.

4. *Nonspecific feedback questions*

   Within this group of questions are the global questions that are asked to determine if students have understood something that they just heard. With specific feedback questions the teacher can find out what is or is not understood rather than asking a diffuse question that does not diagnose the problem and does not foster discussion.

5. *Teacher's ego-stroking*

   Teachers who tend to talk a great deal, and, more importantly, put themselves in the role of the ultimate authority, can inhibit classroom discussions. These are the teachers who do not allow students to expand on their ideas or who do not place value on student observations and thoughts. Eaton et al. (1977) state that although the teacher may not intend to enhance his or her own power, prestige, or control, the outcome of presenting oneself as the authority is the disruption or squelching of thoughtful, risk-taking discussions in the classroom.

6. *Low-level questions*

   Questions designed to elicit factual or informational level answers tend to end a discussion. Questions of a higher level, designed toward more synthesis, analysis, or evaluation, foster discussion because they encourage creative and critical problem solving.

7. *Intrusive questioning*

   Included in this group are questions that go beyond the level of trust or sense of privacy felt by another person. Personal questions, questions that a student is reluctant to answer, and failure to share feelings are all included in this group. A sensitive teacher should avoid such questions when it is evident that a student is uncomfortable responding to them.

8. *Judgmental response to student answers*

   This occurs when the teacher appraises the student's response in a value-laden way and makes personal judgments about the student's response. Students are reluctant to make contributions to a discussion when they feel they might be criticized or embarrassed. In their description of this behavior, Eaton et al. (1977) point out that the hazard of making judgmental responses increases when the teacher does not know the social and cultural context of the learner.

9. *Cutting students off*
   Instead of refocusing the discussion, at times teachers cut off their students by pointing out that a question will be answered later in the course, or there isn't time to consider a specific aspect at this time. Refocusing a discussion in a positive and nonthreatening manner that does not end a discussion is a skill to be achieved.

10. *Creating a powerful emotional atmosphere and then ignoring feelings and responses*
    This occurs when a highly charged environment is created, and the teacher is insensitive to the degree of emotions generated. For example, if students are discussing death and dying and a student wants to express a personal example, if the teacher continues with the theoretical content without acknowledging the emotional aspect, discussion can be stopped.

11. *Hiding behind the role of teacher*
    This is a subtle and elusive characteristic of some teachers that prevents students from seeing their teacher as a genuine human being interested in and responsive to them. Eaton et al. (1977) imply that the mental image the teacher has of herself/himself should be examined and clarified. Teachers who are sensitive to the feedback their students give them can be helped to break their preconceived notion of how teachers should perform with their students.

Careful review of the discussion stoppers described by Eaton et al. (1977) may well give teachers additional insight into how their behavior can inhibit discussion, and it is suggested for reading as a departure point for self-analysis as well as examination of one's own discussion techniques.

A FEW CAUTIONS ABOUT DISCUSSIONS

As with any teaching strategy, discussions must be directed toward the learning objective. If a discussion is pointless, then students are wasting time. If a discussion is dominated by one or a minority of persons, either teacher or students, it becomes a lecture. If students are not prepared for a discussion, they will flounder and pool their ignorance. Students sometimes have negative feelings about seminars because they have had previous unsuccessful experiences with them. The expression, We've been grouped until we're pooped, is heard by students who have experienced unproductive discussions. Seminar leaders can err in two ways— they can be so permissive that the discussion never becomes focused and meaningful, or they can dominate the conversation with their own ideas, thus inhibiting their students.

SUMMARY

In order for a discussion to be a meaningful and valuable learning activity, it must have some guidance. Keeping the contributions germane to the topic is important if the group is to avoid pursuing tangents that are not productive. The instructor's role includes facilitating communications of all the group members, challenging students, identifying when the group needs information to keep it from floundering, creating a climate for free discussion, and summarizing to keep the group to the task.

Above all, it is important for the instructor to be a sensitive observer of the group process and to avoid domination of the group by some students and withdrawal from the group by others. Unfortunately, once a discussion has deteriorated, it is more difficult to renew it than to have attempted preventive measures earlier.

By seeking clarification of issues and allowing minority viewpoints to be expressed, each member's contribution can be appreciated. An environment in which healthy disagreement is permitted helps to bring out divergent opinions. Because the goal is to seek individual students' ideas, the fact that the student has spoken is what should be reinforced, not necessarily what the student has said.

Instructors who are skilled seminar leaders receive rewards. They know the satisfaction to be gained from successful task accomplishment—helping students solve problems together. As with others who are in leadership roles, instructors may suffer anxiety imposed by the possibility of failure, rebuffs in their attempts to lead students, and guilt when students do not achieve to the degree anticipated. It takes much practice to become skilled in the group process. It is an effort well worth making in terms of student outcomes.

10

Teaching Together as a Team

Whereas team teaching is usually referred to in educational literature as a form of school organization, it will be considered in this chapter as a specific teaching strategy. Team teaching exists when two or more teachers with different preparation, abilities, and skills cooperate and share with one another the responsibilities for course planning and teaching and evaluating a group of students. Team teaching is an effort to improve instruction by the reorganization of personnel in teaching. Two or more teachers are given responsibility for all, or a significant part, of the instruction of the same group of students.

GUIDELINES FOR TEAM TEACHING

Anderson (1964) suggests six broad guidelines for team teaching: (1) all team members, including students or student representatives, participate in the formulation of the objectives for the program or course under preparation; (2) all team members participate, at least weekly, in the formulation of the more immediate objectives of instruction; (3) all team members be given at least periodic opportunity to contribute to the specific daily planning of the course; (4) all team members be at least minimally conversant with the specific daily plans of the other team members; (5) all team members should, at least occasionally, carry on teaching functions in the presence of colleagues whose own roles might alternately be to assist, to observe student reaction, and to offer constructive criticism in subsequent discussion; and (6) all team members participate in periodic evaluation of the program or course.

It seems obvious, after studying these guidelines, that the amount of time required by the teaching team to converse with one another and attend to the group processes, as well as have energy left over for students, is a tremendous undertaking. Team teaching does indeed take more time than individual teaching.

ADVANTAGES OF TEAM TEACHING

Team teaching broadens the quality of students' education by exposing them to the knowledge of more than one teacher. It allows the more competent, the more committed, and the more influential teachers to play a more significant role in the lives of more students. Before becoming a member of a team, an individual teacher may have guided the learning activities of a smaller group of students in a "section" of a course. The teacher may have had little direct effect on the decisions and professional performance of students and other colleagues. Team teaching, then, can improve the quality of instruction by giving teachers an opportunity to learn from other team members. The nursing instructor who is especially skilled in teaching can be given an intermediate leadership role that is still a teaching role. As a team leader, this nursing teacher can share skills and insights with colleagues directly, and thus influence other teachers.

Team teaching can provide a way to allow teachers to specialize and retain their expertise in clinical nursing within the philosophy of an integrated nursing program. Instead of teaching a range of disciplines, this teacher may be the one to help students apply general principles of nursing to a specified clinical area. For example, if a group of teachers, teaching as a team, were discussing the care and problems of the immobilized patient, the teacher with special interest in and expertise with children could help students to understand the physiological, psychological, or sociological effects of immobility on different ages of children. Likewise, in sampling the care of immobilized patients, this teacher could concentrate in one clinical area, that of pediatrics, working with different members of the class at different times.

Anderson (1964) points out that, in spite of efforts to provide teachers with supervision and in-service growth opportunities, the typical teacher in the elementary or secondary school is insufficiently prepared in the subject areas and insufficiently proficient in technical aspects of teaching. The same statement can be made of nursing instructors. Under the false label of academic freedom, all kinds of idiosyncratic, unsuitable, or indefensible teaching practices can flourish in schools of nursing. Team teaching's supreme virtue is that it causes teachers to look at themselves and one another both critically and supportively. It provides the opportunity to see alternatives and discover new solutions to old problems.

Kramer (1968), in describing the utilization of team teaching in a baccalaureate nursing program, points out that by breaking teaching strategies into their individual parts, members of a teaching team skillfully blend strengths and personal preferences in teaching to produce an optimum climate for student learnings. Teachers teaching together bring out divergent points of view, thus encouraging students to challenge ideas and perceptions. Members of the team collaborate in the assessment of student learning behavior by systematically observing students during a class session and sharing perceptions of student feedback. The development of teaching strategies that takes place when a course is taught, planned, and evaluated by a group rather than an individual teacher is considered a major advantage. In order to assess this aspect of the effectiveness of the teaching component of team teaching, Kramer (1968) administered a questionnaire to involved students and faculty. The results indicated that both students and faculty were overwhelmingly in favor of being taught (or teaching) by the team approach. Students favored the presentation of varying points of view. They cited as a disadvantage the lack of continuity and internal consistency, which is more often found in a course taught by one instructor. Faculty rated the opportunity to learn from colleagues as beneficial. New teachers stated that the shared teaching responsibility during the orientation period was especially helpful.

Tarpey and Chen (1978) add to the list of advantages of team teaching by including the point that faculty members are able to teach what they are best suited to teach, when, where, and how. They point out that team teaching enables faculty members to improve their own teaching skills when they invite peers to participate in classroom evaluations and share their student evaluations in a constructive way. They also believe that group mastery of teaching skills and instructional planning gives faculty members confidence in teaching various levels of students in undergraduate, graduate, and continuing education programs. Finally, they cite as an advantage the release time from classroom teaching that can be planned for by each instructor to pursue other scholarly activities necessary for growth and promotion within the educational system.

DISADVANTAGES OF TEAM TEACHING

Disadvantages mentioned in Kramer's (1968) study by the teachers included the increased time required for planning and the slowness of the group process. One-half of the experienced teachers stated there was a feeling of loss of individual autonomy in team teaching.

One fear frequently reiterated by teachers is that team teaching results in a uniform or standard approach to the teaching. In order to be effective, team teaching should not only take into account a teacher's subject area expertise, but it should capitalize on individual teaching styles. It is hoped that there will always be room for individual artistry in the college classroom, but to quote Anderson (1964, p. 125), "the artist must possess a defensible art!"

TEAM LEADERSHIP

Specific questions are frequently raised by faculties of nursing contemplating a team-teaching approach. Is leadership necessary in terms of a formally designated leader? It is thought that it is, for several reasons. First, a large amount of time is needed at the beginning of a course when the teachers are becoming a group. If the team were further burdened to choose its own leader, that amount of time would be increased. It is to be remembered that the teaching team is a task-oriented group. Second, they are assisted by someone designated as responsible, to whom members of the group can turn with problems. The administrator of the school of nursing must have someone who can speak for the teaching team. The "administrivia" of the course must be handled—ordering books, placing library books on reserve, communicating clinical faculty needs, and negotiating for facilities with other teachers in the same school and other schools in the area, to name just a few of the chores.

What are the qualifications of the team leader? Who should select the team leader? Deciding on the team leader will depend on the philosophy of the faculty of the school of nursing and its administration. One alternative is that the team leader be appointed by the administration of the school of nursing. Another alternative is that the leader be selected, or elected, by the teaching team. Research on the formal recognition of the leadership role (Raven and French, 1958) suggests that an elected leader is more likely to be perceived as having legitimate power than an appointed one. A combination of the two means of selection can be accomplished by having the teaching team submit two or more names to the nursing school administrator, who makes the final choice. Because the team leader is responsible directly to the nursing school administrator, sound administrative theory would indicate that the administrator of the school have a voice in the selection. However, because the team leader is also the link from the teaching team to administration, the teaching team should also have a voice in the selection and, as indicated above, will accept an elected or partially elected leader more readily. Therefore, the joint decision of both interested groups (teaching team and administration) appears to have advantages.

Some schools of nursing, organized into teaching teams, rotate the team leader. This has the advantage of developing the leadership potential of a large number of teachers, but it can decrease continuity. If the team leader is selected by his or her peers to be a masterful teacher, the rotation of team leader would depend on the particular talents of the other faculty members.

SIZE OF TEAM

Remember the problems relating to group size, as discussed in Chapter 9, when considering the size of the teaching team. It might be advisable to consider dividing a large group of students and teachers into two different teaching teams to avoid the problems of communication that tend to occur with teams that are too large.

Grouping of students and class size are more easily manipulated when team teaching is utilized. By sheer tradition, perhaps, many schools of nursing divide classes into clinical teaching groups numbering from 8 to 10 students, into seminar groups having 20 members, and into large lecture-discussion groups consisting of an entire class. Experience to date seems to indicate that when a faculty first becomes involved in teaching as a team, teachers essentially use the same teaching procedures they did when teaching alone. It is important to keep in mind the advantages and disadvantages of both large and small group teaching; within the limitations of space in the college, the teaching team can develop flexibility in selecting the size of the group and activities to meet the instructional objectives most effectively.

SUMMARY

As Kramer (1968) points out, developing a team approach to teaching is not a simple task, nor is it one that should be contemplated without adequate preparation and planning on the part of the faculty. It requires a faculty group willing to investigate various teaching strategies and ways in which the talents of faculty can best be utilized for the benefit of the students. Tarpey and Chen (1978) aptly discuss the importance of faculty members being willing to share educational philosophy and beliefs about how students learn and their beliefs about nursing. Although the rewards for faculty members who have taken this step toward true collaborative teaching are great in terms of knowing that their students are receiving the advantage of many more ideas and talents than could be given by one teacher, there is no question but that consensus development, the process of becoming a team, and interdependence is time consuming and sometimes frustrating to the faculty members. It cannot be stressed enough that unless faculty can truly develop a commitment to this collaborative way of teaching it may create more problems for both faculty and students than it will solve.

PART 3

STRATEGIES FOR TEACHING INDIVIDUAL STUDENTS

11

Individualizing Instruction

The goal of individualizing instruction has, in recent years, gained increasing acceptance among educators in various fields. Reports appearing in educational and nursing journals attest to the fact that there have been many efforts made toward this goal. Traditional teaching methods are being challenged for several reasons. Among them is the growing awareness of individual differences. There is much evidence to support the theory that each person learns in unique ways, different from every other person. With the wide variety of experiences that occur with maturation, the differences become even greater.

The student population in nursing programs has become increasingly varied. Greater numbers of ethnic minority students, men, and older women are entering nursing. Many students are returning to school after raising a family. Many students have had some previous education or experience in health care that makes them different from the basic nursing student who enters a nursing program directly from high school. Traditional lockstep methods, in which all students in a class are expected to study the same thing at the same time, are no longer adequate to meet the needs of such a heterogeneous group. The challenge facing nursing educators is to adequately respond to the needs of individuals while providing education that is relevant to the needs of society and is adequate to meet the standards of the profession of which they are members.

Although efforts are being made in nursing schools throughout the country, it is clear that the methods used in nursing education are still highly traditional. There is a regular use of common lectures and assignments for groups of students. Rarely are students tested for the purpose of determining which teaching strategies would be best for them or what their perceptual strengths and weaknesses are. Rarely are different media used so that the student can select the ones that are preferred. Rarely are students allowed to take a different route to meet the requirements of a course. Some of the methods that have been instituted in an effort to provide some degree of "individualized" instruction have become traditional in the sense that the methods, such as independent study or learning modules, are required of all students. Whatever method is used, any situation that requires all students to do the same thing at the same time or rate cannot be considered to be responsive to the special needs of individual students (Wilson & Tosti, 1972). The challenge before all of education is no longer equality of educational opportunity but, rather, equality of educational outcome (Bloom, 1980).

This chapter will present three main topics: tools for determining individual learning style, examples of research about learning styles, and characteristics of individualized instruction. The chapter serves as an introduction to individualized instruction and will be followed by three chapters, each discussing one strategy for individualizing instruction.

TOOLS FOR DETERMINING LEARNING STYLE

Learning style refers to the unique ways in which a student perceives, interacts, and responds to a learning situation. Examples of specific tools that can be used to diagnose learning style include:

1. The Learning Styles Inventory by Renzulli and Smith (Ferrell, 1978) is an instrument that can be used to determine student feelings about nine specific learning methods: projects, simulation, drill and recitation, peer teaching, discussion, teaching games, independent study, programmed instruction, and lecture.
2. The Productivity Environmental Preference Survey (PEPS) (Price et al., 1979) is an inventory for the identification of individual adult preferences of conditions in a working and/or learning environment. It takes approximately 15 minutes to complete and investigates 21 categories in four stimulus areas as follows:
   Environmental: Provides information about desired levels of sound,

temperature, and light, and the degree of formality of the physical setting.

Emotional: Gives information about the extent of personal motivation, persistence, responsibility, and amount of structure needed.

Sociological: Yields information about whether a student learns best alone, with peers or pairs, in teams, with adults, or a combination of these.

Physical: Provides information about perceptual strengths—visual, auditory, tactual, or kinesthetic involvement—the need for food/fluid intake, time of day, and need for mobility. The reader is referred to Dunn and Dunn (1978) for more extensive discussion of each of these areas.

3. The Learning Style Inventory (LSI) (Kolb et al., 1971) is a nine-item questionnaire in which the respondent is asked to place four words in the order that best describes personal learning style. Four learning modes are represented: concrete experience, reflective observation, abstract conceptualization, and active experimentation. The LSI takes about 5 minutes to complete (Kirchhoff & Holzemer, 1979).

4. The "cognitive mapping" technique of Joseph Hill (Cross, 1976) has a student take a battery of tests, which are designed to yield a profile of 84 traits that describe that student's learning style. A computer is used to process the test results into a cognitive map to be used in preparing a "personalized educational prescription" (PEP).

RELATED RESEARCH

Dunn and Dunn (1978) claim that there is a wealth of well-conducted research that verifies that each student learns in ways that are different from others. Examples of available research conclusions follow:

1. Students are able to accurately predict the method through which they will learn at a superior level (Dunn & Dunn, 1978).

2. Students who are taught in a method that is in harmony with their learning style score higher on tests than those for whom the method and learning style are not matched (Dunn & Dunn, 1978; Trautman, 1979; Douglas, 1979).

3. Closed-minded students exhibit less tolerance for learning tasks that require a great deal of autonomy (Osborn, 1973; Osborn & Thompson, 1977).

4. Students with a high locus of control are more comfortable in a more structured learning environment (Koop, 1968).
5. Cognitive style is a potent variable in academic choices and development, vocational preferences, interaction strategies used, and processes selected for teaching and learning (Witkin, 1973).
6. Students classified as "dependent" prefer clear directions, while more "internally directed" students assume more responsibility for their own learning (Witkin & Moore, 1974).

The possibilities for research in nursing education settings in the area of learning styles and teaching strategies are great. It seems clear that one method of teaching that is good for all students will not be found. Rather, educators might focus their efforts on developing a variety of strategies and learning alternatives so that each student can select those through which he or she can obtain the most productive learning.

WHAT IS INDIVIDUALIZED INSTRUCTION?

Basically, individualized instruction (II) is the use of teaching approaches that focus on individual learning needs and styles and allow the highest level of achievement by each student. It is a goal that many nursing educators have been working toward for several years, although it is difficult to achieve without major changes in traditional philosophies and procedures. Those interested in moving in the direction of a more individualized approach may gain insight into the requirements of II by looking at its specific characteristics. The following list summarizes the views of several authors (Cross, 1976; Dunn & Dunn, 1978; Forman & Richardson, 1977; Knowles, 1978, Milton, 1975; Flanagan, 1971; Gibbons, 1971; Weisgerber, 1973) in this respect:

1. An II program requires active involvement of the learner and places the responsibility for learning on the student.
2. The teacher in an II program is a facilitator, manager, resource person, and consultant in the total learning process.
3. II requires specification of explicit objectives.
4. Feedback and evaluation are integral parts of II.
5. II is flexible by providing the student considerable choice in selecting from alternative activities and multisensory resources, the sociological pattern to be used, and the pace at which learning will take place.

The Student's Role in Individualized Learning

The role of the student in individualized learning (IL) is one of an active, responsible participant. Active rather than passive involvement of the learner has long been recognized as desirable (Dollard & Miller, 1950; Hilgard, 1956). More recently, Markle (1977, p. 13) stated: "It is not what is presented to the student but what the student is led to do that results in learning." If one believes that learning is a lifetime process and that nursing requires a practitioner who can think and make decisions independently, then active involvement is crucial in the educational preparation of the nurse. While traditional classroom situations encourage the participation of some but not others, individualized programs require the participation of every student.

Active involvement of a student can include either mental or physical processes. The student should be required to participate, recall information, think through problems, and use judgment and reasoning, that is, to be personally involved with the materials for learning. Many examples of active involvement of a learner are available. The list of ideas that follows is particularly pertinent to nursing education. It is given in the hope that it will help each reader generate other ideas that are applicable to individual settings. The student might:

Answer questions about a topic or a printed or mediated clinical situation

Compute problems in drug doses and intravenous rates

Prepare a nursing care plan, drug study, diet plan, or teaching plan

Manipulate equipment, materials, and models

Interview an individual or a family

Work with one or more peers in a particular learning task

Apply material to an actual situation in various clinical settings—hospital, home, clinic, community, and so forth

Role play

Research/investigate available community resources for health care, transportation, or shopping

Demonstrate a procedure

Diagram a process

Collect prepared resources for teaching peers or clients

Produce learning materials for teaching peers or clients

Write reports

Conduct experiments

Play games or complete puzzles

Participate in groups—brainstorming sessions, task groups, panel discussions, and so forth

These and other activities will involve the student directly in the learning process, which may, in turn, increase motivation, interest, and learning productivity. Students who have become accustomed to traditional methods may require guidance and assistance in becoming more active, responsible participants in learning. Thus, some students will, at first, require more structure than others but can progress, if supported and encouraged, to become more actively involved in their own learning.

The Teacher's Role in Individualized Instruction

The role of the teacher in II is drastically different from that of the teacher using traditional methods. The two key components in individualizing instruction are (1) organization of materials and methods to provide the means for learning and (2) determination of whether or not learning has occurred. Thus, the emphasis is on learning rather than teaching, and teachers need to do whatever best contributes to the achievement of that learning.

The role of the teacher in II has been discussed by many authors (Cross, 1976; Burr, 1973; Dunn & Dunn, 1978; Ward & Williams, 1976; Knowles, 1978; Rogers, 1969; Haney & Ullmer, 1975). A review of these resources indicates that the teacher's role is comprised of four general areas: (1) diagnosis and prescription, (2) management and facilitation, (3) evaluation and remediation, and (4) motivation.

Diagnosis and Prescription. In the area of diagnosis and prescription, the teacher is responsible, at times in conjunction with the student, for determining the variance between objectives and the present status of the student. This may be done in a conference or through pretesting and serves as the basis for deciding what is to be learned. The prescription then becomes that which must be done to achieve those objectives that have not already been met.

Management and Facilitation. Once what is to be learned has been established, the teacher manages, facilitates, coordinates, and guides the student in the required learning process. Teacher responsibilities include designing, structuring, and arranging any activities, experiences, or resources that are expected to lead to the desired changes in behavior. This may involve developing instructional materials in a subject area, coordinating activities in the community, leading discussions, having conferences to monitor progress, providing real-life experiences, elaborating on and interpreting experiences, and, for some students, providing structure and direction.

Rogers (1969) was among the first to express the belief that the aim of education is the facilitation of learning. He also identifies the personal relationship between the facilitator and a learner as a critical element that is dependent on the facilitator's possession of three attitudinal qualities: (1) realness and genuineness, (2) nonpossessive caring, trust, and respect, and (3) empathic understanding and sensitive listening.

Evaluation and Remediation.   During and after the various learning activities, it is the teacher's duty to assess progress and evaluate outcomes. This may be done in face-to-face conferences, observations in simulated or real settings, written testing, and so forth. Feedback about progress is given so that students are aware of their standing and what has to be done to achieve learning if any gaps exist between objectives and performance. This function of the teacher is closely related to diagnosis and prescription, except that diagnosis and prescription imply initiation of a new learning sequence while evaluation and remediation occur during and after a learning episode. The reader is also referred to Chapter 1 for a discussion of reinforcement and to the section in this chapter on feedback and evaluation.

Motivation.   Closely related to the role of facilitator and evaluator is the role of motivator. There is general agreement among learning theorists that the learner who is motivated learns more readily than one who is not (Hilgard, 1956). Through the use of various motivational devices, the teacher sets a climate conducive to learning and stimulates the student to learn what is required. The teacher helps a student set goals, assume responsibility, and identify appropriate learning materials. The teacher provides support, encouragement, and praise and establishes a cooperative, friendly environment.

The importance of the personal relationship between the teacher and student has already been noted. Associated with the function of the teacher as motivator is that of serving as role model. Bandura (Knowles, 1978) established the label of "social learning" for the process of imitation and identification associated with role modeling. Through role modeling, the teacher demonstrates the actions and attitudes that a student should imitate. This is a particularly important mechanism for demonstrating desired interpersonal behaviors in nursing and for establishing learning as a lifetime process. By functioning in a "humanist" role along with the other roles in II, the teaching-learning experiences can become more creative, enjoyable, and productive for both the teacher and the student.

Explicit Learning Objectives

A learning sequence that is purported to be individualized requires a clear statement of what the student is to accomplish and how achievement will be measured. In this way, students know exactly what they are accountable for and can go about reaching stated objectives instead of having to guess what the learning requirements are. Only by specifying what is to be learned can the teacher verify when it has been taught (Wilson & Tosti, 1972). Moreover, active involvement is futile unless learners know what it is they are supposed to accomplish (Cross, 1976).

An explicit objective leaves no doubt about its meaning. Vague terms, such as "appreciate" or "understand," should be avoided, and behavioral terms that are observable should be used instead. However, objectives should not be stated in such minute detail that they become overly lengthy and burdensome. A useful guideline is provided by Wilson and Tosti (1972, p. 18):

> The objective should be stated in only enough detail to enable several knowledgeable observers to agree that the observed student behavior represents an adequate accomplishment of the objective.

For example, consider the objective: Describe in 20 words or less what is meant by a physician's order that reads, "NG replacement, ml for ml." Knowledgeable observers would agree that each milliliter of nasogastric tube drainage is to be replaced with 1 milliliter of an ordered intravenous solution.

Just as an explicit learning objective is of benefit to the student so it is also to the teacher. It will help the teacher clarify instructional goals, select or design instructional materials, identify entering and terminal competencies of the student (Glaser, 1968), and evaluate the instructional program itself.

The discussion in this section has focused only on the importance of making objectives explicit. Many other excellent references that discuss types and levels of objectives and provide guidelines for writing objectives are available. Further discussion of objectives in relation to mastery learning will be presented in the next section on feedback and evaluation.

Feedback and Evaluation

It has been shown that any teaching method will be improved by prompting and feedback (Johnson & Johnson, 1975). Individualized instruction requires the establishment of a monitoring and evaluation system for continuous assessment of individual performance. Objective evaluation, based on clearly stated behaviors, helps the learner to develop competence that is expected. Knowledge of results is important so that the student knows when objectives have been achieved or when something else must be done in order to reach them.

The emphasis in individualizing instruction is on the mastery of *all* objectives by *all* students rather than on how well or how poorly objectives are met by students in comparison with one another. Evaluation of a student against stated objectives is called mastery learning, criterion-referenced evaluation, or competency-based evaluation in contrast to normative evaluation, in which students are compared with one another by the use of the "normal curve." In mastery learning, standards are often stated at a minimum performance level; however, a higher level is possible and desirable if educators encourage higher quality performance of all students and allow students to have more time, if needed, in which to achieve objectives. Objectives at varying levels may also be stated if it is necessary, within a particular setting, to designate student performance level by the use of letter grades.

Cross (1976) summarizes research that indicates that the level of achievement in a more traditional curriculum has little to do with success later in life. It is her belief that learning to achieve and to develop one's best talents is more likely to lead to self-fulfillment and, perhaps, success. As described in Chapter 1, learning theorists agree that reward is preferable to punishment for increase in learning. Changing the focus from differential grading to grading based on standards of performance provides students with greater reward and positive reinforcement for continued achievement rather than constant reminders of their relative standing in a group.

Bloom (1968) reports both cognitive and affective gains from the use of mastery learning. He claims that 95 percent of students can attain mastery of most learning tasks if given sufficient time and adequate human and educational resources. In fact, IL is based on this premise. According to Cross (1976) many people mistakenly equate the preservation of the normal curve with the preservation of academic standards. She advances the idea that standards are best served when students learn the material.

In relation to affective gains, Bloom (1968) states that they include the belief that one can attain mastery and competence, a view of oneself as adequate, more positive feeling about the subject, increased cooperation among students, and an increased interest and motivation for learning, both in relation to the subject at hand and lifelong learning. Thorman and Knutson (1977) provide similar results in the areas of attitude toward learning and degree of motivation. Ely and Minars (1973) further corroborate the positive affective outcomes by showing improved scores for students on a self-concept scale after using mastery learning.

When using mastery learning, evaluation is of two types: formative and summative (Bloom, 1968; Airasian, 1971). Formative evaluation is continuous and is used to provide feedback to the student and the teacher regarding the progress toward achievement of objectives. It tells what has been learned and what still needs to be learned. It may be carried out as part of a unit of study or as part of an entire course. It serves, in either case, to help a student move toward the desired competence. If there are areas not yet mastered, the use of formative evaluation provides feedback about those areas. Such a process implies that activities and resources that can help students correct any deficiencies must be readily available for use.

There are different methods for providing ongoing feedback. One involves the use of self-evaluation or peer evaluation of performance using videotaping or criteria check lists. Other possible forms include responding to a clinical situation, answering questions, filling in crossword puzzles, applying past learning to a clinical situation, and responding to attitude scales. The related role of the teacher is to determine what needs to be done next. If the evaluation is part of a clinical experience, the teacher may also provide feedback in the form of written or verbal anecdotal notes. Regardless of the method used, the student should be aware of progress and/or problems at all times and have the opportunity to do what needs to be done to reach objectives. This is in contrast to the inadequate learning that may occur when a student is a member of a large group and does not receive individual feedback or assistance.

As with formative evaluation, summative evaluation provides evidence of learning success or lack of it. However, summative evaluation is carried out at the end of instruction, either in a unit or a course, and is used as final evidence of mastery of stated objectives (Airasian, 1971). Typically, students in traditional courses do not have an opportunity to correct errors or be retested. In mastery learning, if objectives are not reached, the student continues to work until they are.

Summative evaluation shows how students have changed as a result of learning activities and tasks. It may involve the same tools used in formative evaluation or they may be different as long as the behaviors that are part of the learning objectives are reflected. Summative evaluation can include performance in a simulated or clinical setting, participation in group discussions or reports, responses to attitude scales, performance on various types of written exams, or answering questions about a videotaped episode. One technique for helping a student know which objective has not been met is to key each test item to its related objective(s) and learning activities. In this way, the student is able to restudy the area needed and to retest at a later time. This does, of course, require the availability of alternate test forms so that the student actually demonstrates mastery of an objective rather than memorization of a test item.

Flexibility of Student Choice

The provision of choices recognizes the characteristics of adult learners outlined by Knowles (1978). He believes that the maturational process increases the differences among individuals and results in a learner who (1) has a need to be self-directing, (2) is ready to learn those things that will facilitate the fulfillment of social or professional roles, (3) has a broad experience base on which to build new learning, and (4) approaches learning with a problem-centered, life experience orientation.

Three areas in which the student in an individualized learning program should have considerable choice are (1) pacing of study, (2) selecting the sociological pattern to be used, and (3) choosing from among alternative activities and multisensory resources.

Self-Pacing. Pacing has already been mentioned in the previous section on feedback and evaluation by referring to Bloom's view (1968) that 95 percent of students can learn a subject to a high competency level given sufficient time and appropriate help for doing so. Self-paced learning can be defined as that educational method that recognizes that students learn at different rates and encourages/allows the student to use the amount of time needed to reach stated objectives (McBeath et al., 1974).

Just as self-pacing is closely aligned with mastery of stated competencies, it is also closely associated with placing the responsibility for learning on the student (McBeath et al., 1974). One related problem is that a student may not be self-disciplined, motivated, or adept at managing time for learning so that the objectives can be met within a reasonable period of time. Depending on the limitations of time (such as a semester or a year), the teacher can assist a student in dealing with these problems and in making the involvement with self-pacing a positive, growing experience. The teacher provides encouragement, guidelines for the amount of work that should be done by a particular time, orientation about what is expected, and continued interpersonal contact. It is also crucial that the amount of work be realistic for the unit structure and the time period involved. Experience indicates that there are a greater number of lack-of-completion problems when the student in a self-paced course is also taking traditional courses that have definite deadlines and examinations (McBeath et al., 1974). If this situation is unavoidable, it is even more crucial to provide the type of assistance already outlined.

It would be erroneous to conclude that a self-paced course or program is automatically individualized. Other characteristics, referred to in this chapter, must also be present. However, there are some real advantages of self-pacing in and of itself. It allows some students to move more slowly and others to progress more rapidly; it responds to the needs that most students have at some time or other to be absent in the event of unavoidable occurrences, such as illness; it allows students to take time off for financial, physical, or emotional rejuvenation; and it permits scheduling of learning as an important, but not the only, event in one's life.

Although self-pacing in an unlimited period of time is theoretically possible, this presents significant management problems associated with credit for courses; registration and add–drop procedures; determination of student–teacher ratios and teaching loads; and the use of clinical agencies, classrooms, and other resources. It would be worthwhile for those in nursing education to continue to deal with these problems. In spite of them, however, there are many ways to increase the number of self-pacing opportunities in nursing programs. Techniques include the use of independent study, modules, contracts, and computer-assisted/ managed instruction. Independent study will be discussed in the next section, and the specific strategies of learning modules, learning contracts, and computer-assisted instruction will be discussed in Chapters 12, 13, and 14.

Sociological Pattern. Sociological pattern refers to the number and type of people present in a learning situation. The student who has full control over the selection of the sociological pattern to be used for learning can decide whether to work alone, with one or two peers, with a small group, with a larger group, with adults, or with a combination of these. Although such a choice may not be fully realized, in many instances the student can select the pattern to be used. For example, a student who is learning facts about a particular clinical situation may be given a choice of which sociological pattern to use. At other times, when involvement in group or cooperative effort is deemed necessary, the teacher may require the student to work with others. Even then, however, the student may choose with whom to work. As the unit of study is prepared by the teacher, an effort is made to include various options so that the student can either select the favored pattern or understand why a teacher believes that a particular pattern is desirable for a certain objective or group of objectives.

The discussion of types of sociological patterns will take place under two main headings: independent study and learning with others.

Independent study.   Independent study (IS) literally means that a student carries out the activities for learning independently of the teacher. Other terms that may be used synonymously with IS are self-study, self-instruction, self-directed study, and autotutorial study. It is, perhaps, the use of these terms that has led some people to believe that the teacher is uninvolved in the learning process or that the student alone decides what, when, and where to learn. Neither is the case, however. Both teacher and student roles change. Both are involved in a different way than in traditional education. The student has a greater responsibility in all aspects of learning and is more actively involved in deciding what, when, and where to learn and what activities will be completed. However, the teacher who designs or approves the study determines how much flexibility will be allowed. The unit of study may be highly structured, very flexible, or somewhere between the two extremes. Faculty members who have no more to do with the student's experiences after objectives are devised are abdicating their responsibility. Sommerfeld and Hughes (1980, p. 416) believe that student performance in independent experiences "must be carefully developed in much the same way as other well structured learning activities." They go on to say that allowing students complete freedom without holding them accountable is not educationally sound. On the other hand, any study unit that requires all students to use IS entirely or that is so heavily structured that there are no options cannot be called individualized.

Independent study in some form is probably the method most widely used by nursing educators in an attempt to individualize instruction. Early efforts involved students who had special interests and talents that teachers wished to address. Independent study permitted and/or encouraged enriching experiences for those students who wished to go beyond the minimum requirements of a course (Sorensen, 1968). It was generally reserved for the academically superior student who wished to investigate a topic or problem of personal interest.

Progressively, the design of the IS project was seen as a joint effort between the student and teacher. While viewed by Hanson (1974) as an opportunity to promote personal and professional growth, it was pointed out that both the teacher and student must agree on the goals of the study, how student progress will be monitored, how experiences will be recorded, and amount of supervision the instructor will provide.

The concept of self-directed study is now widely accepted among nursing educators. IS is often mentioned in nursing literature as a central strategy used for basic nursing education (Langford, 1972; Stein et al., 1972; Thompson, 1972; Wittkopf, 1972; Beyers et al., 1972; Blechert et al., 1975; Honey, 1975; Cudney, 1976; Layton, 1975; Rochin & Thompson, 1975; Blatchley et al., 1978; Jones & Kerwin, 1978). Others discuss IS in relation to inservice education and continuing education (Reinhart, 1977; Huntsman & Thompson, 1977; Schmidt, 1977; Sherer & Thompson, 1978; Smith, 1980). In fact, IS is the basic sociological pattern required with learning modules, learning contracts, and computer assisted instruction.

From the reports it is clear that there are definite values to the use of IS. Besides increasing student responsibility and participation, IS allows for differences in student needs, interests, and learning rates. It permits students to study required content at a time that is most appropriate to a particular clinical setting and most convenient for them. IS units help to establish a minimal level of knowledge in a particular subject that is required of all students, provide enrichment experiences for some students, and allow some students to move more rapidly through learning experiences. IS materials are particularly helpful in providing background and preparation information to a student preparing for a specific clinical experience. In this way, teachers and students have more time for clinical practice, the quality of the clinical practice is improved, and discussions on the application of content to client needs can take place. Further, IS cultivates the skills and attitudes that are essential to lifelong learning and provides practice in analyzing, evaluating, and using information.

Learning with others.   Just as students should be given the option of learning independently at times, so should they be provided opportunities to learn with others. Nursing is a profession that requires the effective use of interpersonal skills and the ability to work cooperatively with others. The instructional sequence, then, should provide options in the type of social environment to be used in order, first, to provide more individualized learning and, second, to provide social interaction that will facilitate the development of skills for working effectively with others.

The involvement in a social situation may be an end in itself for those who need human warmth and support in order to function and learn effectively. It is known that social situations offer highly effective learning experiences (Cross, 1976). Specific support for the value of learning with others is offered by Knowles (1978) in his discussion of adult learners. He states that the maturing adult, by having participated in many previous experiences, is a rich resource for learning through the use of such experiential techniques as discussions, laboratory, simulation, field experience, team projects, and other action-oriented techniques. Consequently, nursing educators should provide such experiences and, in addition to rewarding independent thought and action, foster and reward the student's involvement in cooperative interaction with others.

There are many positive aspects of learning with others. The list that follows is not an exhaustive one but is given in an effort to enumerate some of the benefits of social interaction during learning. Learning with others:

1. Fosters cooperative effort and democratic participation
2. Prevents isolation of the learner
3. Increases motivation and interest
4. Enhances the development of analytical and problem-solving skills
5. Provides practice in development of ideas
6. Facilitates the development of interpersonal skills
7. Increases sense of responsibility for shared learning
8. Broadens exposure to others' ideas and ways of thinking
9. Increases confidence of the individual
10. Broadens knowledge base through collective participation
11. Provides practice in integrating information from varied sources

The two main forms for individualized learning with others are pairs and small groups. Research evidence indicates that students who desire "close, friendly interpersonal relations develop problem-solving skills better when they are assigned to work on the problems in pairs . . ." and that "weak students are especially likely to profit from peer tutoring" (Cross, 1976, p. 125). Furthermore, those students who are uncomfortable in teacher- or authority-dominated situations profit from learning with their peers (Dunn & Dunn, 1978).

Several arrangements of peers working together in learning situations can be found in the literature. Each of these seems to support the notion that mutual learning is more productive for some students and that teaching something to a peer is an excellent way to increase one's own understanding. McKay (1980) describes a peer group counseling model in which peers are used as support persons. In this method, students are trained to provide listening, support, and interaction with the primary goal of enhancing problem-solving skills of the person being counseled. DiMinno and Thompson (1980) report on the use of an interactional support group for graduate nursing students.

Several examples of the use of peer teaching or evaluation are available. The proctor-managed system and the peer-proctor system are described by Wilson and Tosti (1972). In the proctor-managed system, a student who is more advanced than the proctored student provides a supporting role and gives feedback and evaluation of learning at specified points in the learning sequence. Their scope of responsibility is well defined, with the authority to evaluate student performance (rather than teach) and to indicate to the student what the next assignment should be. On the other hand, the peer-proctor system uses either an advanced student or one who is presently enrolled in the course to work with an assigned group of students or to be "on duty" at certain times to serve all students who need help. Another variation of the same system is to select proctors on a rotating basis in relation to which students are able to complete a particular unit of study most quickly. In the peer-proctor system described, student proctors work for either credit, bonus points, or pay.

Rochin and Thompson (1975) report on a variation of the peer-proctor system in a nursing education setting. They described the use of student "facilitators" who work for either credit or pay and who dispense learning materials for student use in a learning center, grade module posttests, and provide assistance with learning in relation to assigned learning modules.

Several authors discuss the value of peer teaching for the development of skills needed in the future practice of nursing. Burnside (1971) believes that assigning a student to supervise another student in the clinical setting increases autonomous functioning and helps the student develop teaching behaviors, expand resources for learning, and obtain feedback about behaviors. Clark (1978) believes that student interaction with one another as student, teacher, and peer helps to prepare them for future experiences with peer review. Boguslawski and Judkins (1971) state that the opportunity for peer observation and counseling is an important factor in the development of independence and creativity.

There are other, less formal, ways to pair students for learning. In a particular unit of study the student may be given the option or may be directed to work with a peer. This method is particularly useful in a basic skills course so that each student will have a partner with whom to work, try out ideas and techniques, and provide mutual feedback about performance of the skills. A student can also be encouraged to work with another student in answering a specific set of questions, generating ideas about dealing with a certain clinical situation, or doing research on a particular topic. Ways to encourage peer interaction and learning in the clinical arena include dual assignments, having one student serve as "helper" on a rotating basis to three or four other students, or assigning a student at least one time during a clinical rotation to work as a "free agent" and become involved in a variety of activities that may not be possible with a regular assignment. Each of these is useful at different times to increase peer interaction, enhance the use of limited clinical facilities, and allow the student to function in different roles.

In addition to learning in pairs, small-group techniques are helpful for achieving the positive results of learning with others already listed on page 139. It is crucial that nursing students learn to work effectively as members and leaders of groups in situations that are reality oriented (Clark, 1978). Only by having such experiences can the students, upon graduation, be expected to assume those roles in their work and community lives. The use of small groups has been one of the most pronounced trends in educational practice during the last 2 decades (Knowles, 1978). Small-group involvement is thought to provide interpersonal benefits through interaction with peers and to help students grasp complex ideas and relate more effectively to subject matter (Phillips, 1973).

A small group is usually made up of five to nine people and may work in either a formal classroom setting or in other, less structured settings. When a specific learning assignment is involved, it may be one that has been designed by the teacher alone, the teacher and students together, or students alone. Learning activities often include individual or collective reading or viewing; the use of case studies, critical incidents, or situations; consideration of a particular problem; answering questions; or development of a care or teaching plan.

Three types of small-group techniques that seem particularly helpful to learning in nursing will be summarized. They are supportive, teaching, and task groups (Clark, 1978). The supportive group is usually an informal one in which students select one another when they have mutual needs. However, the peer-counseling model by McKay (1980) also had support as one function with upperclass students trained as peer counselors. Both formal and informal groups can be helpful in decreasing the level of stress of nursing students so that energies can be used more productively for learning. In addition, the peer-counseling model can be used as the training ground for students who are learning to lead groups and developing counseling skills; thus, for the student in the group it is a supportive group and for the student serving as counselor it is a teaching group.

The task group and teaching group are the major types with which formal education is concerned. In general, all group work used in education has some elements of both teaching and task since students are involved in completing some type of task assignment in order to achieve certain knowledge and skills. Therefore, there will be no attempt to differentiate between the two types of groups except to make a few comments specific to task groups that are not true of the usual teaching groups.

The primary purpose of small-group or team learning is to involve the members of the group in a cooperative effort to learn about a particular topic that is of interest to all members of the group. The group members often serve as catalysts to each others' ideas so that combined learning is increased. As an added benefit, the students gain knowledge about group dynamics.

Although any small-group work may be thought to be involved in the completion of a task, there are some unique characteristics of "task groups." Participants are organized around a particular task only for the duration of the specific job to be done; leadership evolves and changes depending on the strengths of individual members at different times; and members participate equally in some portion of the task (Bevis, 1978). In addition, much of the work of the task group can be carried out individually or in pairs and then brought back to the total group for presentation, consolidation, and agreement. Thus, each member has a particular job that is important to the work of the total group. Any member who does not complete a subtask interferes with the accomplishment of the primary task for which the group is responsible.

There are a number of ways in which task groups can be used in the educational process. A few possibilities are listed below:

1. Demographic study of a community
2. Research on various aspects of a selected topic, such as child abuse
3. Preparation of an annotated bibliography on a topic
4. Investigation of problems of particular groups, such as housing, transportation, medical care, and recreation for the elderly

Regardless of the procedure for small-group work that is used, it is important for the teacher to meet certain responsibilities in order to increase the chance for group effectiveness. A clear goal or task must be established; real and meaningful problems that stimulate interest must be selected; guidelines for group operation must be provided; expectations of group participation and activity must be clarified; required resources for group work must be accessible; and constructive feedback must be given. Furthermore, the teacher should remember to give options for independent and paired learning in addition to group learning when a specific sociological pattern is not a requirement of the activity.

Alternative Activities and Multisensory Resources

The term "media" includes all resources used in a learning sequence to help the student achieve stated objectives. When there is a combination of several communication media, the term, multimedia, is used.

Diversity of learning style in relation to type of media is well recognized (Ward & Williams, 1976). Some people learn best through the written word and reading; others through spoken instruction and hearing; others through visual presentation and seeing; and some by handling concrete forms. For many, learning is enhanced with a combination of two or more media forms. Table 11-1 includes examples of media appropriate to nursing education in relation to the four main learning modes: reading, seeing, listening, and manipulating.

Table 11-1
Learning Modes, Formats, and Representative Examples of Media

Learning Mode	Medium Format	Representative Examples of Media
Reading	Print materials	Textbooks, reference books, charts, pamphlets, outlines, workbooks and studyguides, handouts, crossword puzzles, printed programmed instruction, journals, newspapers, scripts
Seeing	Pictorial materials, visual representations	Filmstrips, filmloops, videotapes, television, 8-mm and 16-mm films, displays, exhibits, posters, photographs, slides, overhead transparencies, diagrams, cartoons, simulated activities, demonstrations, flow charts, graphs, sketches
Listening	Auditory	Lectures, seminars, paired and small-group discussions, skits, audio and videotapes, one-to-one interaction with teacher, peer, or client, oral presentations, panel discussions, debates, simulations
Manipulating	Tactile, kinesthetic	Practicing with real or simulated items, lab activities, manipulating or constructing models, playing games, drawing, filling in worksheets or workbooks, preparing bulletin boards, charts, graphs, or displays

Learning activities must include a variety of media so that people who learn best in a particular way can use their preferred method. Individualized instruction presumes the availability of alternate routes to reaching the objectives (Dirr, 1976). Whether or not the use of media improves instruction and increases individualization depends on how media forms are used in the instructional sequence. To be effective, media should not be merely attached to traditional instructional procedures (Dirr, 1976) simply for the sake of using media. Rather, each learning resource should be selected because it is believed to be the most useful for achievement of instructional goals. At times, several different types of learning resources may be equally appropriate.

An important role of the teacher is the use of a variety of methods so that each student is able to choose one that is personally most productive for reaching objectives. The degree of individualization increases when the student is provided with options about learning activities to be completed and type of resources to be used. Secondarily, student attitude toward learning will be improved since there is a greater degree of control over the learning situation (Ward & Williams, 1976). At the same time, learning productivity is increased since perceptual strengths are supported.

If there are several ways to present the same subject matter and exposure to each way would result in extensive repetition, it is undesirable to require that a student use all media forms. Rather, the teacher should determine what alternatives are possible and allow each student some choice among the different media. The choice might be between a reading activity in a textbook or journal and a viewing/listening activity using a filmstrip and audiocassette. Too often students have no choice—a list of learning resources is given and students are instructed to study everything. This may occur because the teacher feels that, otherwise, "something will be missed." It may be because objectives are not yet well enough defined in relation to the topic for a particular level of student. Thus, it is easier to require students to complete all related activities than to specify objectives to reflect exactly what is expected of the student.

There are valid reasons why the degree of flexibility of student choice is restricted at times. Desired experiences and available resources may be limited due to overcrowding of clinical facilities, lack of fiscal resources to purchase or develop media, or lack of quality or availability of commercial media. In such situations, it may still be possible to allow individual choice through the creative use of those resources that are available. A few examples follow: (1) reporting on a topic in written, verbal, visual, or auditory form or a combination of these; (2) writing personal learning objectives for an experience; (3) attending a lecture or completing a guided, independent learning activity (such as a module or audiotutorial lesson); (4) selection of a client with whom to complete an interview, carry out some type of physical or developmental assessment, or apply prior learning; (5) selection of one or more peers with whom to work on an activity or project; (6) selection of one topic from a list of several on which to report to a group; (7) deciding level of mastery in relation to desired grade (contracting to do a specified amount and quality of work for a specific grade); and (8) choosing from among two or three optional plans for how to complete a learning experience or project.

When it is not possible to provide choices, every effort should be made to use activities and resources that are multisensory. In this way, the perceptual strengths of the student can, at least, be accommodated for a portion of the learning experience, and each medium helps to reinforce another. For example, if there is a filmstrip/audiocassette and a chapter in a text that discusses different aspects of a topic, the student might be required to study both but would achieve greater gains using the medium that is preferred. Learning can be increased in the non-preferred medium if it can be supplemented with teacher-developed materials that focus or direct student learning. One example of the latter would be the preparation of a study guide or an audiotape to be used by a student in combination with the required media.

Another example, in a motor skill area, is when the student is learning to thread intravenous tubing through an infusion pump and put the pump into operation. The best learning result would probably occur through a combination of several activities—reading the procedure, seeing a demonstration, seeing a diagram of proper threading, and, finally, manipulating the tubing and the pump. Further, typical problems may be simulated in a controlled setting so that the student has an opportunity, in a safe environment, to learn to deal with them. It is easy to visualize the difference in level of clinical performance between a student who has participated in all of these and a student who has had an opportunity only to read the procedure and see a demonstration.

There has been no attempt made in this chapter to discuss which medium is best in different situations. The reader is referred to some excellent references that do so (Kemp, 1977; Price, 1971; Diamond, 1977).

SUMMARY

This chapter included a general discussion of individualizing instruction as background for the specific strategies to be discussed in the next chapters. Several examples of tools that can be used to determine learning style were included. The conclusions of a few research studies in the area of learning style were given. The major emphasis, however, has been on discussing the five major characteristics of individualized instruction: (1) student actively involved and responsible for own learning; (2) teacher is a facilitator, manager, resource person, and consultant; (3) objectives are explicit; (4) feedback and evaluation are incorporated; and (5) flexibility of student choice in relation to pacing, sociological pattern, and activities and resources. There has been an effort throughout to give examples that are applicable to nursing.

12

Developing and Using Modules for Instruction

One strategy by which mastery learning and individualization can be achieved is the learning module. In the past decade, the use of modules for teaching a variety of subjects at all educational levels has been described in educational literature. In fact, Cross (1976, p. 75) credits the learning module with being at the heart of an "instructional revolution" in which the accent is on learning. Previously, Novak (1973, p. 4) had observed: "The use of some form of modular instruction is probably the fastest-growing trend in the history of Western education." Three surveys support these conclusions in relation to community colleges in general and to associate and baccalaureate degree nurse education programs. In a survey of community colleges (Cross, 1976), almost three-fourths of the respondents reported some use of learning modules. A survey of associate and baccalaureate degree nursing programs (Thompson, 1980) revealed that almost two-thirds of the respondents were using modules or learning packages in their programs. And in a later survey of baccalaureate nursing programs (Knippers, 1981), 76 percent of the respondents indicated that modules and packages were used in some courses. Also, there are many reports in the literature that describe the use of learning or other closely related strategies for nursing education at the undergraduate, graduate, and postgraduate levels. Some of these will be cited throughout this chapter.

A problem that confronts anyone who wants to gain a historical perspective of utilization of learning modules is that a variety of terms are used to describe essentially the same approach. One of the earliest educational uses of the term module was in 1971 by Craeger and Murray. Others who have used the term since include Russell (1974), Rochin and Thompson (1975), Cross (1976), Shute (1976), and Swendsen, Meleis, and Hourigan (1977). Some other terms, used during the same period, to describe approaches reflecting characteristics shared with learning modules are Minicourse (Postlethwait & Russell, 1971); Audio-Tutorial Package (McDonald & Dodge, 1971); Individualized Study Unit (Lewis, J., 1971); Learning Packet (Ubben, 1971; Ward & Williams, 1976; Ray & Clark, 1977); Learning Activity Package (Cardarelli, 1972; Layton, 1975; Brock, 1978); Interactive Learning Package (O'Connor & Jones, 1975); Contract Activity Package (Dunn & Dunn, 1972); Individualized Instruction Package (Duane, 1973); Individualized Learning Package (Freeman et al., 1975); and Individualized Learning Unit (Magidson, 1976). Blatchley, Herzog, and Russell (1978) used the terms module and minicourse synonymously. The term module will be used throughout this chapter since we believe it is a more inclusive and descriptive term.

WHAT IS A LEARNING MODULE?

The learning module, a strategy for individualizing instruction, is a self-contained instructional unit that focuses on a single concept or topic with a few well-defined objectives. Although other instructional formats may be (and should be) incorporated, independent study is at the center of the use of learning modules. Through independent study, the student has increased control over when and where learning will take place. At the same time, a learning module should reflect other characteristics typical of individualized instruction (II) as given in Chapter 11.

The design of a learning module determines the degree to which the learning situation is individualized. Design depends on the philosophy and expertise of the developer, specific concept or topic of the module, and availability of learning resources for use with the module. The finished product should demonstrate a close integration of the individual components of instruction—objectives, strategies, and evaluation. This is most likely to occur when one uses a systematic approach while developing a learning module. One such approach is described by Thompson (1978), the steps of which are paraphrased below:

1. Select a topic and describe its general purpose or intent.
2. Outline the pertinent characteristics of the student group that will use the module.

3. List learning objectives and complete a task analysis to determine what tasks a student must perform to reach objectives.

4. Identify content pertinent to each behavioral objective.

5. Develop learning activities for each objective.

6. Select or develop media (all materials) to present the content and allow variations in learning style.

7. Validate instructional media and techniques with content and/or instructional experts.

8. Develop tools for testing and evaluation to reflect each objective.

9. List any required prerequisites.

10. Identify and arrange for any necessary support services.

11. Develop the guide that the student will use for completion of the module.

12. Develop a tool for feedback from the student about the module.

13. Use the module in a trial run with a student group.

14. Make necessary revisions.

Elements of a Learning Module

What does a module look like? An outline of typical components of a learning module is given below:

1. Table of contents

2. Introduction, including purpose, terminal objective, and general directions

3. List of prerequisites and suggested resources

4. Instructional objectives

5. Pretest

6. Resources

7. Activities

8. Self-checks of progress

9. Posttest

10. Feedback on module

Each of these components will be discussed briefly. The reader is also referred to the sample module included at the end of this chapter for an illustration of each of the elements (Appendix 1).

Table of Contents.   If the printed packet of the module is more than a few pages long it is helpful to have a table of contents to identify each section and its page location. This allows the student to find a section quickly and easily with minimal confusion and frustration. A table of contents is especially helpful for the student who has already had an introduction to the subject covered by the module and who wants to locate the objectives and the pretest to decide if the module or parts of the module have been previously mastered. A table of contents is also useful for the student who wants to review the list of resources to be used so that what is required and where it is located can be determined ahead of time. In this way, time for study of the module can be planned and organized more productively. Furthermore, a table of contents aids the student in locating a particular activity or section when self-check or posttest results indicate the need to do further studying in order to achieve mastery.

Introduction. The introductory section of the module lets the student know the purpose of the module, the significance of study of the material covered, the terminal objective, and how best to advance through the module. The language should be directed to the student and written at a level that the student can understand. In this section, as in others, every effort should be made to avoid typographical and grammatical errors that distract or hamper progress of the student.

Prerequisites and Suggested Resources. A list of the prerequisite knowledge and skills is given so that students are able to determine if they have the background necessary for success with the module. Prerequisites are best stated in specific behavioral terms so that the student can understand more clearly the required entry behavior for module study. A list of suggested resources is useful for the student who needs to make up deficiencies before beginning study of the module. Notice in the sample module that alternative resources are given. This allows the student more flexibility in selecting which resource to use.

A prerequisite test and key can be included to help the student make a quick self-assessment of desired knowledge and skills and indicate the direction that review should take, if needed. Bloom (1980) suggests that teachers should pay greater attention to entry characteristics of the student. He believes that what a student brings to a course may have more to do with achievement than the course itself. Thus, greater gains can be assured in a particular learning situation if the student is first brought to the desired level of achievement on prerequisites for that learning task.

Instructional Objectives. Well-defined learning objectives specific to the module are stated so that expectations are clear to the student. As stated in the definition of learning module, only a *few* objectives should be included. Although the actual number depends on specific content, it is preferable if the number is limited to 15 or less per module. If more than 15 objectives are necessary for a particular topic, the developer of the module should consider narrowing the topic further so that fewer objectives will be covered in the module. For example, this may require that modules be developed on two subtopics rather than one module on one major topic.

Objectives should, when possible, require more than simple recall and involve the student in using the content in a practical learning situation. The objectives should be relevant to the experiences of the student and the goals of the course in which the module is used. They should be matched precisely with module content, resources, activities, and items for evaluation and testing. In some cases, each objective is listed separately with directions and a list of resources and activities specific to that objective given immediately after the objective. In other cases, all objectives for the module are given and resources and activities keyed to each objective. The latter is the format used for the objectives in the sample module.

Pretest. A pretest representing all learning objectives should be a part of every module. Length of the pretest will vary depending on the level of complexity of the objectives and the type of activity required to demonstrate mastery. However, if the objectives are few and well defined as specified in the definition, a pretest representative of all objectives would not be lengthy. A maximum time period of 15 to 30 minutes is recommended. This does not seem unreasonable when one considers that traditional testing usually involves the use of a 1-hour examination to cover lectures, readings, and so forth for one-third to one-half of a semester or quarter. The difference is that the objectives for a module are more delineated so that the student knows exactly what is expected and can, thus, be expected to reach each objective.

The pretest is primarily a mechanism for assessing prior knowledge and skills to determine if a student must complete all, part, or none of the activities of the module. For the student with previous exposure to the module subject area, success on part or all of the pretest serves as positive reinforcement and recognition of that learning. It is possible, then, to give credit for previous learning and allow the student to progress more rapidly through required learning experiences. The pretest thus represents a point at which decisions about prior mastery or nonmastery are made. For the student who demonstrates nonmastery of all or part of the module, either the total module or selected parts of a

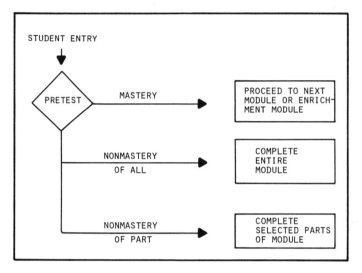

Figure 12-1
The pretest as a decision point in module use.

module can be completed based on exact pretest results. Figure 12-1 depicts the pretest as a decision point and shows the possibilities indicated by pretest results.

The pretest also serves other functions that are useful to the learning process. By providing a preview of what is in the module, it "sets the scene" so that the student knows what to expect. In addition, since it tests the same objectives, the pretest gives an indication of what the posttest will look like. Because of this, the pretest may be used, if desired, as an alternate form of the posttest or as a self-evaluation tool by the student to determine readiness to take the posttest.

The key for the pretest can be included in the module for the student to use independently for self-assessment or self-evaluation. However, if the student is to be given formal credit for prior learning, it is probably necessary for the teacher or an assistant to retain the test key and review pretest results personally. If performance of a skill is involved, the student may demonstrate competence in several ways. The student may perform the skill in front of an observer with a criteria checklist or may do a private videotaping of skill performance for later review by an evaluator. The latter provides greater flexibility to the student and the teacher and can decrease the amount of stress that the student feels in the testing situation.

Notice that the format of the pretest in the sample module includes a notation with each question telling which objective is being tested. In this way a student with prior learning is able to determine more easily which activities can be skipped and which ones must be completed. A key provides immediate feedback about level of knowledge if the pretest is being used independently by the student. The key can be placed immediately after the pretest in the module or at the end of the module with other keys to self-checks and the posttest. The key can also be provided in other than written forms, such as on an audiocassette tape, for the student who prefers to listen or who gains more from listening and reading at the same time.

Resources.   A list of alternative or required resources must be given so that the student will be directed to materials to be used in the achievement of objectives. Alternate resources from which the student may choose increase student options to select preferred materials. When such alternatives are given, it is important that each provides equal access to achievement of objectives. One alternative may be a visual and auditory experience using a filmstrip and audiocassette or a videotape. Another may be a reading activity in a textbook or journal. Another may have the student handling and manipulating real objects or models. One important advantage to giving a choice of resources is that limited resources or those housed in a learning center are used more efficiently when a number of students need the resources at the same time. If alternatives cannot be given, it is important to use a variety of multisensory resources so that, at least, different perceptual strengths are addressed during a learning experience. Such variety also helps to increase motivation and maintain interest.

A listing of resources also indicates if there are limitations in their availability. For example, a module that requires the use of a videotape would necessitate the presence of the student in a learning center or viewing area. On the other hand, a module that requires the use of a textbook owned by the student can be completed wherever and whenever the student chooses. A module that directs the student to discuss a particular topic in a small group cannot be completed without the availability of a group. In all of these instances if the student is aware, in advance, of such limitations or special requirements, the student will be able to plan time for study of the module more effectively. Student frustration will thus be decreased since the student will not begin study of a module only to discover that an important resource is not readily available.

Self-Containment.   A module is self-contained since it is made up of everything that is required to reach the objectives and to measure their achievement. Self-containment can take two forms: (1) all module components are under one cover or in one package that is portable, and (2) the module is made up partially of peripheral components that are not easily transportable. When all module components are in one package, access and convenience to the student are increased. For example, in a module on the topic of Clinitest urine testing, everything required can be contained in a small carton. Such a module is usable either in a learning center or skills laboratory or, if sufficient kits are available, may be transported to any location selected by the student. Often, as in this case, portability is easily accomplished by the use of kits containing practice supplies to be checked out by the student. When such kits are involved, it is important for someone to be available and responsible to check them out to the student and to check and replenish the contents when returned.

Portability can also be achieved by synthesizing material from various resources and putting the information under one cover—the all print module. This type of module, however, has some distinct disadvantages. First, it is only in print and may not be the best type of learning experience for many students. Secondly, it requires greater time for development and is more difficult to revise and update than one using peripheral resources that can be readily deleted or added.

In some cases, portability is increased by using easily transported equipment and materials for checkout. For example, a compact filmstrip-viewing and audiocassette playback unit and a copy of a filmstrip and audiocassette program available for checkout broaden accessibility and add to the convenience of the student. An arrangement of this type requires ample equipment and materials as well as personnel for their dispensing and servicing. It is also crucial that some understanding be reached and communicated about replacement or repair of lost or damaged items.

Portability is difficult or impossible to achieve in many instances: when heavy or expensive equipment is involved; when form or cost limits availability of media resources; or when location of required resources is specialized, as in a clinical setting or the community. In such cases, self-containment at a specific location is the only alternative. For example, a module that requires the use of a computer, specialized medical equipment, or media of which there are limited copies would necessarily require completion where those resources are located. This is restricting to the student in one sense because the student must go where the resources are—often in a learning center or skills laboratory with limited hours of operation. If this is required, it is of primary importance that adequate hours are scheduled so that learning requirements can be achieved within a reasonable period especially if time for completion is limited. Although operating hours may be limited, the student still has some options: selecting a personally convenient time within specified hours, deciding which resources to use if alternatives are stated, and choosing whether to work alone or with a friend.

Activities.   Learning activities that direct the student's use of the resources focus the student's efforts on the objectives to be mastered and give the student practice in reaching objectives. Directions provided with each activity must be clear so that the student is able to use time productively and avoid unnecessary confusion. Activities should reflect the type of action specified in the objectives and involve the learner in active participation with the content. Participation can take the form of mental, written, interactive, or manipulative exercises and can involve the use of study questions, guided reading, worksheets, projects, charts, diagrams, puzzles, simulated or actual clinical experiences, practice with models or actual items, interaction with others, and so forth. As stated previously, activities may be indicated with each objective in turn or each activity can be keyed, as in the sample module, to indicate which objective it relates to.

Some activities are required of all students. This is particularly true when resources are limited, or different resources are not comparable. Even when students are completing the same activity, they may be given an option of which medium to use when the content among the various media is similar. It is desirable, when possible, to use alternative activities to allow some choice by the student. The choice could be either to complete a short paper on a particular topic or to give a 5-minute speech on that topic to a group or on an audiocassette. Another choice could be to select which drug or clinical situation will be used for more in-depth research. The possibilities are limited only by the availability of resources and the creativity of the person designing the learning experience.

Some activities are completed by only a few students for the purpose of enrichment when a student is able and interested in studying a topic to a greater depth. They may be designed by the student, by the teacher, or by both. When modules are used in conventional grading situations, enrichment activities are often used to differentiate among the various grade levels.

Self-Checks of Progress.   Self-evaluation checkpoints are included to provide immediate feedback to the student about progress toward meeting each learning objective. They let the student know if an objective has been reached; if not, the student is directed to repeat an activity, do an alternate activity, or seek counseling from the teacher. Figure 12-2 illus-

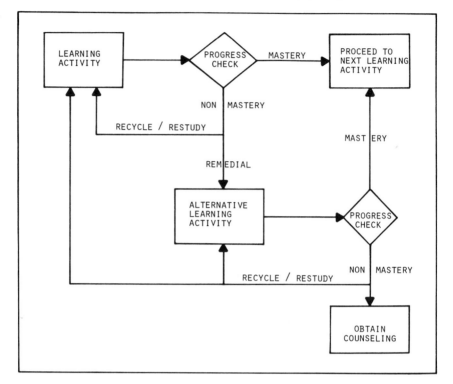

Figure 12-2
The progress self-check as a decision point and alternative routes indicated by self-check results. Adapted from Wilson & Tosti, 1972, pp. 138–139. Used with permission of Individual Learning Systems, Inc., P. O. Box 225447, Dallas, Texas 75265.

trates the use of the self-check as a decision point in the learning module and shows different routes that the student can take depending on self-evaluation results.

The self-check also serves secondary purposes by indicating readiness for the posttest and giving the student clues about what the posttest will be like. Self-checks may be similar in form to pretest and posttest items or may have a different form as long as learning objectives are clearly reflected.

Posttest.   A posttest is used to determine whether or not the student has achieved mastery of the learning objectives stated in the module. As with the pretest, the posttest covers all objectives, has notations to indicate which objective is being tested, and is of comparable length. If posttest

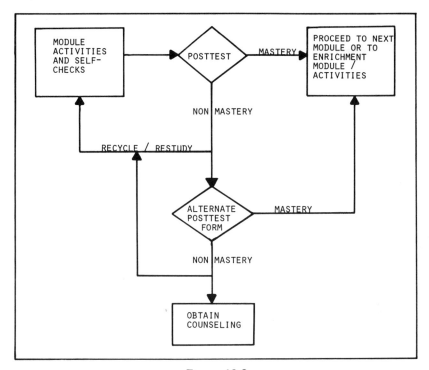

Figure 12-3
The posttest as a decision point, with alternative routes indicated by posttest results.
Adapted from Wilson & Tosti, 1972, p. 140. Used with permission of Individual
Learning Systems, Inc., P. O. Box 225447, Dallas, Texas 75265.

results indicate that objectives have been met, the student can proceed to
another module or learning experience. If objectives are not met, the
student must repeat activities or do alternate activities in order to
achieve what is required. Figure 12-3 shows the posttest as a decision
point in the module and shows the different routes for achievement of
mastery.

The posttest is used by the student, the teacher, a teacher's assistant,
or a computer to provide data to indicate what the next learning experience should be or the need for restudy of material. If used by the
student alone, the posttest is often a part of the printed module packet.
If it is to be graded by someone other than the student, the posttest
is usually retained by the teacher or an assistant or generated by a computer.

Posttest items, like the pretest and self-check items, can take various forms—multiple-choice, fill-in, short answer, true-false, essay, performance—depending on the content and level of objective. It is desirable, when possible, to use test forms other than written. For example, diagrams, slides, videotaped situations, and exhibits offer testing variations that increase interest, capitalize on different perceptual strengths, and add realism. Also as with the pretest, posttest items are keyed to indicate the objective that each item is related to so that a student can restudy those sections associated with a missed question.

The pretest and the posttest can be the same, especially if the teacher wishes to determine exact gains from module study. Broader evaluation might be accomplished, however, if the two tests are different. Alternate forms of the posttest are needed when retesting on a module is required. The pretest, if different, serves as one alternate form, or a computer can be used to generate alternate test forms. In addition, the teacher who maintains a file of questions related to each objective will be able to construct an alternate posttest, if necessary.

Posttest results, in addition to indicating mastery or nonmastery of objectives, provide feedback about effectiveness of module design. If a number of students study a module and the posttest confirms that they have met the objectives, posttest items are validated and the design of the module is supported. If, on the other hand, nonmastery is evident, it is necessary to analyze the posttest and module design to determine what revisions are needed. The objectives may need to be rewritten. Resources and activities may be inappropriate. Posttest items may not adequately reflect the objectives. Whatever the case, analyzing posttest results provides data that help a teacher to make alterations that will add to the effectiveness of the learning module.

Feedback on the Learning Module. Students may be requested, usually on a voluntary basis, to give their impressions about each module used. They may be asked to write out general impressions or be given a tool that will direct their attention to certain important aspects for evaluation. Student feedback provides information from the student's perspective that is helpful for making revisions in the learning module. The sample module includes one example of a feedback form for use by students (see page 190).

Utilization of Learning Modules

The learning module represents an instructional *system*, since it involves an integrated assembly of components (resources, activities, equipment,

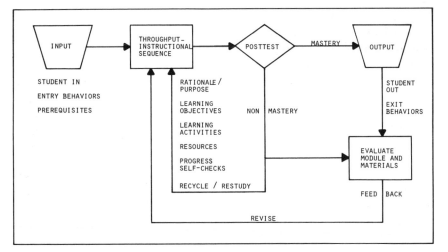

Figure 12-4
A modular system (Russell, 1974; Herrscher & Baker, 1969; Wilson & Tosti, 1972).

people) that operate in organized interaction to transmit instructional messages designed for achievement of predetermined objectives and provide feedback about effectiveness of the system. Figure 12-4 depicts an operational diagram of the modular instructional system. Such systems can be used on a small scale to provide independent study options and enrichment or on a large scale to teach an entire course or all courses in a curriculum.

Common Uses.   Learning modules can be used to teach any subject in any setting, including schools, places of employment, and the home. They can be designed for formal credit, continuing education, self-improvement, hobbies, or other uses. In education, they are a mechanism for individualizing instruction and serve to extend the influence of a teacher over a greater number of students and to take advantage of the contributions of experts on a particular topic. Russell (1974, p. 96) identifies the more common uses of modules as "regular instruction, enrichment, remedial instruction, establishing entry behavior, absentee instruction and correspondence courses." Russell's list will be modified somewhat and applied to situations in nursing education.

Regular instruction and absentee instruction.   Modules can be used to provide regular instruction in part of a course, an entire course, or all courses in a curriculum. Most of the reports in the literature in the last

10 years describing the use of modules (or other self-instructional learning packages) show that they have been used for regular instruction of selected courses or the total curriculum. The most common application of modules to regular courses is for teaching basic technical and physical assessment skills. Nursing programs using modules for this purpose include the Intercollegiate Center for Nursing Education, Spokane, Washington (Ray & Clark, 1977); San Jose State University, California (Rochin & Thompson, 1975); University of California, San Francisco (Swendsen et al., 1977); and the University of Washington, Seattle (Sullivan et al., 1977).

At San Jose State University, California, modules are used to provide regular instruction to all students in more than half of the courses in the baccalaureate nursing major. It is the predominant teaching strategy in two, 2-academic unit, sequential basic skills courses. Each course covers 1 semester and focuses on preventive and therapeutic nursing measures for assessing, maintaining, and restoring human functioning. Although each course is limited by the semester and the student is responsible for completing designated modules each week, there are many opportunities for selection of preferred media, pacing of study within each week, and choice of whether to study and practice alone or with one or more peers.

Each week's modules involve independent study; independent, paired, or small-group study and practice; and large-group discussion. Each module has activities that are to be completed by the student at any time before a scheduled practice lab and a full group session on the topic. These activities can be done independently or with one or more peers, as desired by the individual student. Some module activities require the use of audiovisual media, textbooks, journal articles, or other references that are located in the Nursing Learning Resource Center (NLRC) in the Department of Nursing, which is open from 8:00 a.m. to 5:00 p.m., Monday through Friday. Other activities require textbooks, handouts, and equipment that each student owns. Some modules have alternate resources from which the student selects based on personal preference or access.

The scheduled practice lab, 3 hours in length, is attended by 18 to 20 students (one-third of total group) and is staffed by a regular faculty member and a skills laboratory coordinator who has a master's degree in nursing. This lab provides an opportunity for students to practice designated skills, ask questions, seek clarification, and obtain feedback about performance of skills. The skills are practiced in small groups, pairs, or independently. There is considerable flexibility that allows a student to attend another lab period or to use the skills laboratory independently to practice or obtain assistance from the skills lab coordinator. There are approximately 22 hours each week during which the skills laboratory is open but unscheduled. Students are encouraged to use that time to increase self-confidence and proficiency in performance of skills before use in the clinical setting. Many students who have completed the two courses also return to the NLRC and the skills laboratory to review or practice skills that they anticipate performing during the next week in the clinical area or community.

Following the practice lab, a 50-minute discussion period with the total group is scheduled in a regular classroom with the faculty member. This time is used to discuss general concepts related to the skills that have been studied and practiced, answer questions, clarify, and assist the students in applying what has been learned to practical situations. All students usually attend these; however, the discussion is recorded on audiocassette and placed in the NLRC for independent student use if a class is missed or review is desired.

Each module has a pretest, self-checks, and a posttest with keys for use by the student for self-evaluation. A technique used for self-check or testing is the "criteria sheet" outlining key points related to performance of each skill. Table 12-1 shows one example of a criteria sheet.

A total of 300 points is possible in each course. There are 100 points divided between two practical examinations made up of exhibits or problems about which the student must answer questions, make decisions, calculate problems, carry out some action, and so forth. Responses consist of short answer or item selection and are written on an answer sheet identifying by number each exhibit or problem. There are also 100 points divided between two written examinations given during the scheduled discussion periods. These tests contain 50 questions—usually multiple-choice, matching, or true-false—for which the student selects one answer per question. Item analysis and scoring of the written tests are done by computer. The third 100 points are gained through performance on five written and five practical quizzes at intervals throughout the semester. For the latter, the student is assigned a skill to perform or selects a card, from among five or six possibilities, that tells the student which skill to perform. A teacher observing each student's performance uses a criteria sheet to evaluate and determine points gained.

Students are notified at the beginning of each course how many points are needed to make a certain grade. Thus, the student is able to work to achieve maximum points possible rather than competing with peers. This grading system also encourages students to help one another and participate in supportive feedback about performance of skills. Although some may view it as "grade inflation," the increased clarity of

Table 12-1
Sample Criteria Sheet Used in Skills Course at
San Jose State University, California

Administration of medication via heparin lock

_____ Prepare syringe with normal saline (amount depends on number of medications being given); use as small a gauge needle as possible.

_____ Prepare syringe with heparin flush (standard heparin lock holds 0.5 ml).

_____ Prepare medication in proper dilution.

_____ Make sure all air is out of syringes.

_____ Label each syringe, unless readily recognizable.

_____ Observe site for inflammation; if none, proceed.

_____ Cleanse injection port with alcohol sponge with firm circular motion.

_____ Stabilize injection site and insert needle of NS syringe being careful not to penetrate tubing.

_____ Aspirate for blood return to check for placement of needle in vein.

_____ Flush lock with 2 ml NS to clear out heparin; observe site for infiltration; determine if patient experiences burning or pain.

_____ Detach syringe from needle; maintain sterility of syringe by adding sterile needle.

_____ Attach syringe with medication to needle and inject medication at a rate appropriate to the drug while observing the patient for adverse reactions; detach syringe from needle.*

_____ Reattach NS syringe to needle and flush lock with 2 ml NS to clear out medication; detach syringe from needle.

_____ Attach syringe with heparin to needle and fill lock with weak heparin solution; withdraw needle from injection port.

*Note: Intermittent medications can also be given via the heparin lock and an IV line with a volume control chamber. In this case the IV tubing would be attached to the needle at this point and allowed to run at an appropriate rate.

learning expectations accomplished through modules and the precise knowledge of what must be accomplished for each grade have resulted in an approximate grade range in the skills courses as follows: 59–65 percent "A", 33–38 percent "B", 2–3 percent "C", and 0–1 percent "D" or "F".

Modules are also used for teaching theoretical foundations courses at San Jose State University, California (Rochin & Thompson, 1975); as an option for independent study in regular nursing courses at the University of Illinois Medical Center, Chicago (Layton, 1975); and for medical and/or surgical nursing courses at Ohio State University, Columbus (Collart, 1973) and Purdue University, Indiana, associate degree program (Blatchley et al., 1978). In addition there have been some reports of totally modularized curriculums in nursing, including West Valley College, Saratoga, California (Rose & Riegert, 1976); Evanston Hospital

School of Nursing, Illinois (Beyers et al., 1972); the associate degree program for licensed practical nurses at the Southern Illinois Collegiate Common Market (Ferrell, 1978); and the self-paced nursing curriculum at Florida State University, Tallahassee (Cowart & Burge, 1979).

Modules can also provide regular instruction when students are absent from regular classes due to illness, transportation problems, family circumstances, and so forth. Thus, the student is able to complete work that could not be done at the regular time. Access to modules for independent study prevents a student from being forced to drop out, take an "incomplete," or fail because of unpreventable inability to attend classes. In addition, for the student who does get an "incomplete" when course work has been satisfactory but unfinished, the teacher may specify certain modules to be completed at mastery level so that a grade for a course can be recorded.

Enrichment.   Modules can be used to provide an expanded, in-depth learning experience beyond the basic essential requirements for all students. Such experiences are enrichment opportunities for the student who is motivated or interested in pursuing a topic further or wishes to gain points or credit toward a higher grade. Russell (1974, p. 116) and Duane (1973, p. 172) refer to these as "quests" while Ward and Williams (1976, p. 32) use the label "DO-ITS" (acronym for Depth Opportunities-Individual Tasks).

Regardless of what they are called, enrichment activities or modules provide an opportunity for individual investigation and creativity beyond the basic performance-oriented learning exercises. Enrichment can be achieved by providing optional activities as part of a module, by having separate, optional modules from which the student selects, or by allowing a student to design a learning experience related to a particular topic. When the optional activities are attached to the module, they are usually directly related to module content but provide an opportunity to apply the knowledge or skills gained from the basic module in new and different ways. Optional activities should be meaningful to student experiences and appropriate to the level of the student so that interest is maintained and student time is used productively. Optional activities that are incorporated into a module for enrichment purposes can include:

Write a paper related to some aspect of the topic. (Length and number and type of references might be specified.)

Construct two learning aids to be used for client/peer teaching.

Prepare a short speech to deliver to peer group.

Prepare a demonstration of a skill.

Create a game or puzzle for teaching clients/peers.

If separate, optional modules are used, they are usually at least indirectly related to the basic learning experiences. Optional modules are often on specialized topics or issues that go beyond what can be included in the basic curriculum. The types of activities included should encourage projects or creative productions that require in-depth investigation and application of knowledge. Optional modules can include:

Complete research on a particular topic or on people and places associated with the topic.

Complete a survey of newspaper articles, magazine articles, and television reports relevant to a particular topic.

Prepare slides, tapes, posters, or bulletin boards that can be displayed or used by other people.

Interview a public official, members of a profession, or a client.

Locate and abstract three or four journal articles per week related to topics under weekly discussion.

Write a reaction paper to television specials, movies, or books associated with the topic being studied.

When the student is allowed to select a topic and design an enrichment activity, the teacher requires that the student prepare, in advance, and obtain approval for the plan of action, questions to be answered, type and number of resources to be used, and method of reporting. Teacher supervision is needed to provide necessary guidance and assure that the finished product is of the desired quality.

Ideas for enrichment activities may be generated by the teacher or the student by thinking about experiences that are interesting and rewarding to them. The teacher may also consider the various aspects of topics for which there is not enough time in the basic curriculum and talk to other professionals about topics and issues or students about their interests and personal goals. Specialized topics or issues are particularly appropriate. A few examples are:

Moral or ethical issues, such as abortion, genetic engineering, right-to-die, and pollution of air, water, food.

Professional issues, such as entry into practice, credentialing, standards of practice, and compulsory membership in professional associations.

Social issues, such as crime prevention, segregation, welfare, overpopulation, rent control, child or spousal abuse, and rape.

Special topics, such as genetic counseling, use of play with the hospitalized child, reactions of parents to the hospitalization of a child,
compliance with immunization requirements or prescribed drugs, and
client knowledge about side effects of drugs.

Remedial instruction and establishing entry behavior.   These two uses are
closely related in process. Modules can be used for remedial instruction
when a student needs to review content covered previously for application to some current situation. For example, the student in a clinical
course who is having some problem with dose calculation, remembering
pertinent growth and development characteristics, or recalling needed
physiological concepts can either repeat modules used before or use
modules designed specifically for remedial purposes. Although remedial in nature, such modules help establish the desired entry behaviors
for a particular learning experience. Other modules designed for either
or both purposes include a basic math computation module to determine if the student has the math skills necessary to master dose calculation skills, a module on basic research terminology or statistics to determine readiness for a graduate level applied research class, or a module
on the physiology of glucose metabolism in preparation for study of
diabetes mellitus. When modules of this nature are available, students
can be expected to use them to develop necessary entry behaviors so that
it is not necessary to devote limited class time to deal with material
associated with course or topic prerequisites. Those who have fulfilled
the necessary prerequisites are not required to use the modules; others
can use them for review, if desired; and others can make up deficiencies resulting from a lack of earlier education or insufficient recall of
content.

One example of the use of modules for establishing desired entry
characteristics is given by Chinn and Hunt (1975) in graduate level child
nursing instruction at Texas Women's University, Dallas. Module pretests were used in that setting to determine a student's entry level of
knowledge and skills and the results used to direct the learning experiences of the student. If the student lacked basic cognitive and performance skills in ambulatory child nursing, self-directed learning modules
were used to provide a mechanism whereby these skills could be
achieved before attempting advanced work in the clinical specialty.

Assessing prior knowledge for advanced placement.   Although related to
the use of modules for establishing desired entry behaviors, assessing
prior knowledge for advanced placement implies that the student has
had previous course work or experience that may allow skipping of part

or all of a course. Module pretests and posttests, or a sampling of test items, are used to assess individual ability and recognize previous learning. As a result, credit is given and the student placed at the proper level in the curriculum. This is particularly appropriate to determine if any part of a planned program can be eliminated for students with acknowledged previous experience—military hospital corps personnel, nursing assistants, licensed practical/vocational nurses, or registered nurses who have either a diploma or associate degree and are enrolled in a baccalaureate degree program.

Providing nontraditional options for continuing education and degrees. There are several areas of need for educational opportunities beyond the basic nursing program. Among them are (1) many states now require or plan to require continuing education for relicensure of registered nurses; (2) large numbers of nurses desire courses for self-development or increase in professional status through upward mobility; and (3) there is a continuing information explosion.

In nursing, traditional forms of education have not been effective in meeting the needs of the nurse who is employed full time, has family responsibilities, and lives at a distance from educational institutions. Nontraditional methods, such as the learning module, help to provide independent and/or part-time study and flexible scheduling in a setting that is more readily accessible to the home or work setting of an employed nurse.

Home study courses using modules are advertised in professional journals and newspapers. Study materials in modular form are now available commercially.* Such materials are useful for independent study at various levels of nursing education, including continuing education and staff development. When used in a hospital inservice/staff development setting, modules provide increased access to educational materials, broaden learning opportunities, decrease the scheduling and management problems for groups who need the same instruction, and decrease per employee costs of instruction. For example, all new employees can be oriented to the agency through a modularized program that has been developed to incorporate the special characteristics and needs of the agency. Nurses in a clinical unit can be given specialized instruction peculiar to that unit through the use of modules that are

---

*Learning materials in modular form are advertised by Addison-Wesley Publishing Company, Inc., Menlo Park, California; John Wiley and Sons, Inc., New York; AVC Nursing Series, Novato, California; and Mark-Maris Publishers, Buffalo, New York.

completed at home, in the unit, in a learning center, or a combination of these.

Huntsman and Thompson (1977) and Sherer and Thompson (1978) report on the use of modular learning for staff development at El Camino Hospital, Mountain View, California. It is their contention that the program achieves the advantages cited above and frees the staff development instructor to develop quality materials and spend time in the clinical units assessing and validating skills rather than planning, conducting, and repeating formal classes. Essential to this plan is the identification of learning needs by the head nurse and staff member involved and the subsequent independent use of the learning center by the staff member to study materials related to performance expectations.

According to another report by Schmidt (1977), self-paced instructional materials were used in staff development at Presbyterian Hospital, Columbia-Presbyterian Medical Center, New York City. In that setting, a modular curriculum was designed for teaching 15 subject areas common to seven different intensive care units. The intent was to increase accessibility, reduce costs, and improve learning efficiency by means of immediate application in the clinical area. The author also stated an added benefit of allowing the clinical specialist to be more directly involved in patient care and supervision of staff members' clinical performance.

Formalized nontraditional programs used for credit toward a degree include the "extended" or "outreach"* and the "external" degree programs.† In outreach type programs, learning modules are used to broaden availability of learning materials and to increase accessibility to courses for credit in underserved areas. Representative of such programs is the Community Outreach Option that is being developed by the Department of Nursing at San Jose State University, California. Two satellite centers, within the service area but at some distance from the campus, are being set up for use by employed RN students who are preparing for exams for credit or completing the last two semesters of the requirements for the baccalaureate degree. The materials are com-

---

*An extended or outreach program is one providing courses toward the completion of a degree and established by a recognized educational institution in a satellite location convenient to learners' homes or work settings. Course offerings are of the same educational quality as those on campus, lead to the same credit, and are under the direction of faculty with regular appointments (McGill & Molinaro, 1978).

†An external degree program is a program sponsored by an educational institution in which work and life experiences and credit by examination are emphasized, and time for completion is de-emphasized (Brower, 1979; Lenburg, 1976).

pletely modularized and cover the same content as courses given on campus.

Other examples of extended programs include those at both baccalaureate and master's level. The Medical College of Georgia School of Nursing operates satellite programs at both levels (White & Lee, 1977). The University of California School of Nursing at San Francisco piloted an extended master's program on a university campus of the California State University and Colleges System, which had a baccalaureate program but did not have a master's program in nursing (Leveck, 1975). The University of Texas School of Nursing, San Antonio, established outreach centers for continuing education of nurses in underserved areas of South Texas (McGill and Molinaro, 1978; Shockley, 1981). Although only one of the programs (Leveck, 1975) cited the use of modules, this teaching/learning strategy is the major technique currently available to expand educational opportunities for continuing education and advanced degrees.

The best known program of the external degree type is that offered for associate and baccalaureate degrees by the New York Regents. The programs are for assessment only, rather than instructional, using both written and clinical performance examinations (Lenburg, 1976). Although examinations were originally offered in New York State only, assessment centers are now available in other areas of the country as well.

Another program established to provide greater flexibility and individualization and expand educational opportunities for registered nurses is the statewide baccalaureate nursing program established by The Consortium of the California State University and Colleges (Dumke, 1980). As with the New York Regents program, the student decides how and where to obtain course work and practical experiences to achieve desired competencies. However, the California program, in addition, offers a formal instructional program using modules as one option (The Bachelor of Science in Nursing, 1981).

Patterns of Module Use

The patterns of module use in a course or curriculum depend on several factors, including specific material, complexity of subject matter, and level of student. The patterns that will be discussed are time scheduling, subject matter sequencing, sociological format, and grading.

Time Scheduling. Time scheduling for module use falls into two general types, self-paced and specific scheduling. If fully self-paced, the student is given a list showing any required and alternative modules related to the course or the experience and allowed to complete them, including the necessary tests for competency, at a personally determined rate. The grade assigned is either one of mastery or a specific letter grade, depending on the type of course in which the modules are used. The structure for credit can be units per module, units for a certain number of modules within a course, or units for the course in which modules are used. For example, the faculty may decide that a particular module is worth a given amount of credit, such as $\frac{1}{4}$ unit, $\frac{1}{2}$ unit, or 1 unit, depending on the amount of work and complexity of the module. Two or more modules could be combined and given a specified amount of credit, such as 1 unit, upon completion. Or all the modules used in a course can be collectively assigned a certain amount of credit, such as 3, 4, or 5 units. At the present time, the most common pattern is one in which designated modules are used in a particular course, and the student receives credit upon successful completion of *all* the modules

The same general pattern applies as well to specific scheduling, except that modules must be completed within a certain period of time. Modules can be assigned on a weekly basis or, when more flexibility is possible, a series of modules can be assigned to be completed within a certain period of time. That period of time might be 2 weeks, a month, or a quarter or semester. Specific deadlines are necessary when open time patterns are not possible within traditional settings and testing must be done for all students in a course on a fixed schedule (e.g., midterm and final exams). At times, a fixed schedule is also necessary to help those students who are unaccustomed or unable to set their own timetables of completion. In a course with specific scheduling, the student who does not complete the designated work can receive an "incomplete" with the commitment to finish the required work within a designated time period in order to receive a grade for the course. Usually, the student is required to have completed a majority of the course at a satisfactory level in order for an "incomplete" to be assigned.

Subject Matter. The other pattern of module use relates to the sequencing of the modules themselves. The exact pattern depends on the determination of levels of complexity, structure of the curriculum or individual course, and interrelationships among subject areas. Usually the sequencing is established within a particular course or area of study. Basic patterns of module sequencing include single, serial, satellite, and

1. SINGLE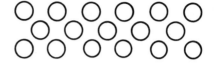

2. SERIAL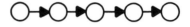

3. SATELLITE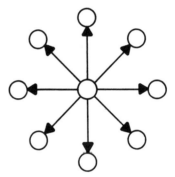

4. STRATIFIED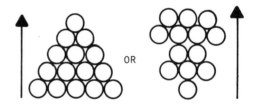

Figure 12-5
Basic patterns of module sequencing. Adapted from Bevis, Em Olivia: Curriculum Building in Nursing, ed. 2, St. Louis, 1978, The C. V. Mosby Co. Used by permission.

stratified (Figure 12-5). Arrows indicate the sequence for study of the modules within each pattern.

Single modules are those that stand entirely alone. They are totally independent of other modules to be studied since they are not prerequisites to other modules nor do they require other modules as prerequisites. Modules in this pattern can be used in any order by students, thus allowing the student to select according to individual needs or preferences. Modules of this type can be used in a clinical course in which available experiences determine which modules need to be studied.

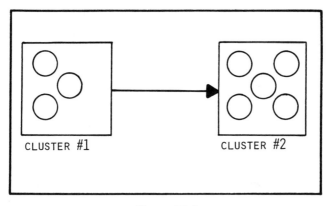

Figure 12-6
Clusters of related single modules, with cluster 1 as prerequisite to cluster 2.

Single modules within a course are usually of a similar level of complexity. Increased complexity is attained with other single modules in succeeding levels of the curriculum. A modification of this pattern, in order to achieve increased complexity using single modules within a course, is accomplished by two clusters of single modules with one cluster prerequisite to the other (Figure 12-6). Modules within each cluster are completed in any order; however, all modules in cluster 1 are completed as a prerequisite to beginning any of the modules in cluster 2.

Modules used in a serial pattern include those that are joined together in a row and that must be completed consecutively. Serial modules are content related, with each one serving as a prerequisite to the next one in the series. It is expected that the farther along a module is placed in a series, the more complex it is in comparison to earlier modules.

Modules in a satellite pattern are those that are joined by commonalities of content, perhaps an introductory or core module followed by several related, single modules that are completed in any order. Satellite modules vary in number, depending on the needs of the specific subject area. One example of material suitable for use in modules in a satellite pattern is shock, when the core module discusses shock syndrome and introduces various shock types and four single modules discuss the types of shock—hematogenic, cardiogenic, neurogenic, and vasogenic—individually.

Stratified modules are those arranged in layers with all modules in each layer prerequisites to the modules in the next layer. Each layer represents a higher level of complexity than the previous layer. Modules at each level are completed in any order, at times, or completed serially,

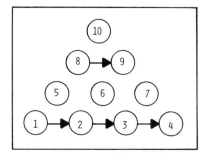

Figure 12-7
Stratified pattern incorporating both single and serial modules.

at other times. Figure 12-7 shows stratified modules using both single and serial sequencing at different levels. Modules 1–4 are serial and must be completed in numerical order. Modules 5–7 are single and can be studied in any order. Modules 8 and 9 are serial with 8 preceding 9. Module 10 is single but must be done after all the rest.

Collectively, achievement of the objectives of all modules leads to attainment of objectives for a total course, while completion of all courses leads to the terminal objectives for the curriculum. Courses may utilize a combination of these patterns of sequencing. For example, modules in one course may be patterned as shown in Figure 12-8. Many other variations are possible, depending on specific material being taught.

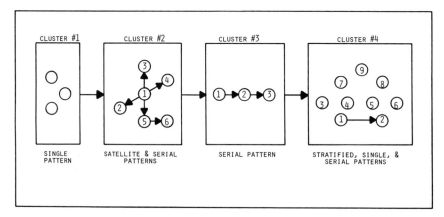

Figure 12-8
Combination of patterns within an individual course.

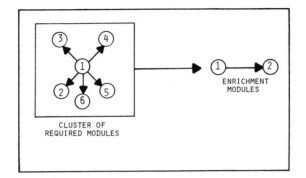

Figure 12-9
Enrichment modules attached to a cluster of required modules.

There are 21 modules in the course shown in Figure 12-8. The modules are arranged in four clusters that are themselves in a serial order indicating that modules in each cluster must be completed before beginning any of the modules in the next cluster. Cluster 1 is made up of three single modules to be completed in any order. Cluster 2 has six modules in two patterns: satellite and serial. Module 1 must be done first; modules 2–5 may be completed in any order; and module 6 must be done after module 5. Modules 5 and 6 could be completed before modules 2–4, if desired. Cluster 3 has three modules in a serial pattern to be completed in numerical order. Cluster 4 is made up of nine modules in a stratified pattern, basically, but also incorporates single and serial patterns. This combination of patterns has already been seen in Figure 12-7.

The modules in the various patterns can have their own enrichment activities as part of each module or additional enrichment modules may be designated. For example, single enrichment modules to be done at any time, depending on needs and interests of the student, can be available or they can be attached to a cluster of related modules as shown in Figure 12-9. The modules in the cluster are required of all students, while the modules outside the cluster can be completed as desired by individual students. One student may decide to do neither of the enrichment modules; another may complete one only—in this case module 1 since it is prerequisite to module 2; and another may decide to do both.

Sociological Format.   As stated previously, the primary sociological pattern used with learning modules is independent study (IS). This provides several advantages. IS allows the student to make some of the decisions about where and when to study. It also provides flexibility for a student who wants to repeat difficult activities or move more rapidly through a module. Efforts should be made, however, to include activities that increase motivation and enjoyment for the student who learns best when involved with other people. Students should be encouraged to work with others when a complex learning task or situation is involved. If the goal of a module is to stimulate cooperative effort and problem solving, the student can be directed to participate with peers in companion or small-group activities such as data collection, brainstorming, or role playing.

The "people" component of the modular system (besides the student and peers) is also very important. Planned student–teacher interaction is crucial. The teacher must be available to answer questions, evaluate progress, diagnose learning needs, and prescribe learning requirements as well as to counsel, encourage, and motivate. This can be done on either a one-to-one or group basis and involve free discussion, questioning, testing, or observation of performance. It is possible to use auxiliary personnel to assist the teacher in these functions. For example, a baccalaureate prepared nurse, an undergraduate student, or a graduate student can observe student practice, grade quizzes, provide feedback about progress, keep records, or refer the student to the teacher when needed. People serving in this capacity are often referred to as "facilitators" (Rochin & Thompson, 1975), "proctors" (Wilson & Tosti, 1972), or "peer tutors" (Keller & Sherman, 1974) and are expected to have mastered the material covered in each module so that they are able to help the students more effectively.

The extent and special needs of each modular program determine the requirements for support personnel. Clerks may be used to dispense and return learning materials to their proper locations, restock disposable materials as needed, assist students with minor problems with equipment or media, keep records of frequency of use of print and nonprint learning resources, and keep records of the number of students using specialized areas such as learning centers or skills laboratories. The record keeping role is particularly helpful for obtaining data needed to calculate costs per student and provide support to budgetary requests for personnel, facilities, equipment, audiovisual materials, and so forth.

When activities require the use of audiovisual or other specialized equipment, it is important that someone, such as a media technician or teaching assistant, be available to orient the students to its use and assist with special problems that occur with media or equipment. A media technician should be available to service audiovisual equipment and materials promptly, in order to decrease down time that affects the learning process. A media technician also assists faculty with development and production of audiovisual learning resources.

The ready availability of learning materials also depends on having a secretary who is responsible for typing modules, cataloging various learning resources, ordering commercial materials, and having printed materials duplicated. When the use of modules or the number of support personnel is limited, it may be necessary to train one person to fill several positions in the basic operation of a learning center. If the one person is a secretary or clerk, it is vital to maintain a close working relationship with those personnel who provide services for equipment maintenance and repair, production of learning resources, and other specialized services.

Grading.   The normal curve has been used for grading for such a long time that current practices are still heavily influenced by it (Russell, 1974). Some educators believe that there must always be a certain percentage of students who fail and that only a few students will be able to learn at a high level.

Bloom, Hastings, and Madaus (1971, p. 45), in their discussion of mastery learning, made the following statement about the normal curve:

> There is nothing sacred about the normal curve. It is the distribution most appropriate to chance and random activity. Education is a purposeful activity, and we seek to have the students learn what we have to teach. If we are effective in our instruction, the distribution of achievement should be very different from the normal curve. In fact, we may even insist that our educational efforts have been *unsuccessful* to the extent that the distribution of achievement approximates the normal distribution.

If one follows Bloom's philosophy, the majority of students, given enough time and adequate resources and assistance, would be able to achieve a high level of learning. Thus, if performance objectives and criteria of evaluation are clearly established for each module, and they are stated at a high level of learning, each student is able to work toward mastery of what is specified. Ideally, then, the grade is simply one of mastery with successful completion or nonmastery when additional work is needed. The formal grade recorded in this situation might be *M* for mastery, *P* for pass, *Cr* for credit, or *A* for excellence.

In actual practice, because of the influence of the normal curve, various grading patterns are seen. Several grading practices that illustrate a compromise between individualized and traditional approaches are outlined below. In general, they represent an attempt to provide some degree of individualization within the established educational structure. No attempt will be made to judge the quality or limitations of a particular grading system.

1. Objectives for modules are stated at a minimal, or *C*, level. The formal grade recorded upon successful completion of required modules might be *C*, representing achievement of the minimal objectives, *M* for mastery, *P* for pass, or *Cr* for credit. If provisions are made for higher grades, the student who desires a higher grade than *C* is required to complete enrichment activities, special projects, or additional modules for extra credit. One example of the use of modules for grade differentiation is when one series of modules must be completed for a grade of *C*, another series for a grade of *B*, and a third series for a grade of *A*.

2. Objectives for individual modules are stated so that those to be completed for each grade are specified. There may also be modules treating the same content area that are developed at different levels—one module with *C* objectives, one with *B* objectives, and one with *A* objectives—from which the student selects depending on the grade desired.

3. A certain number of modules to be completed at a satisfactory level are specified for each grade level. For example, in a course with 10 modules, the grading pattern might be as follows: (a) six or fewer modules completed satisfactorily, a grade of *D*, *F*, or *Incomplete;* (b) with seven, a grade of *C;* (c) with eight, a grade of *B;* and (d) with nine or 10, a grade of *A*.

4. Module posttests are used for self-evaluation only with other tests covering module content given at specified intervals. Students are required to take all tests and to have a grade assigned based on the number of points received from those possible. For example, using total possible points the range for each letter grade is established, and a student knows ahead of time how many points must be attained for a certain grade.

5. A variation of item 4 is that tests over module content are given at specified intervals and the student is required to take a certain number of the tests as well as achieve a certain number of points for each grade level. A student who takes fewer than the minimum number of tests or receives less than the minimum points receives an *Incomplete*, *D*, or *F*, depending on whether or not opportunities for further work exist.

6. Modules are used as one teaching strategy among others, such as lectures. The module is used for preparation for the lecture and the posttest of the module is used for self-evaluation only. The grade for the course is determined by performance on traditional course exams at specified intervals. The grade for an individual student represents the student's relative position in a normative grouping.

Problems Associated With Modular Learning

There are certain problems about which one should be aware when considering or beginning the use of modules in an instructional program. Some of these have been mentioned throughout the chapter. The

Table 12-2

Potential Problems Associated With Student Role and Possible Interventions for Dealing With Problems

Problems	Possible Interventions

Student procrastination related to inability to manage self-paced study.
 	
  Lack of prior experience
  Taking modular course along with traditional course with rigid schedules, requirements, grading
	1. Provide thorough orientation to IS
	2. Set up a suggested schedule for pacing of completion of modules
	3. Begin with modules that are short and relatively easy to complete
	4. Make modules as interesting as possible
	5. Maintain contact with student for support, encouragement, assessment of progress, and assistance, when needed
	6. Use modules in a more structured format at first
	7. Provide positive evidence of success
	8. Schedule quizzes and tests on module content at intervals

Insufficient learning related to failiure of student to assume responsibility for own learning and to choose resources that increase learning effectiveness.
 	
  Access to materials
  Prior experience in traditional courses that convinces the student that high level of learning is not attainable
  Using modules in a traditional course with a definite schedule regardless of level of mastery
	1. Maintain contact with student for assessment of progress and assistance when needed
	2. Set up evaluation/testing sessions so that student is made aware of problem areas/need for further practice
	3. State objectives at a high level (traditional B or A level) and increase flexibility of time for practice and repetition
	4. Devise ways to demonstrate increased learning quality that is possible with mastery learning
	5. Include reality application experience as part of module so that importance of learning is demonstrated
	6. Increase portability of learning materials and maintain as extensive hours as possible in practice labs and learning centers

Feeling of depersonalization by student related to the change in student and teacher roles.	1. Maintain face-to-face contact with student through conferences, seminars, personal appointments 2. Incorporate peer, small-group, and large-group interaction into modules 3. Provide personal attention as indicated by student need/progress

Table 12-3

Potential Problems Associated With Teacher Role and Learning Resources and Possible Interventions for Dealing With Problems

Problems	Possible Interventions
Poor teacher acceptance related to change in teacher role, lack of recognition of value of mastery learning, and lack of rewards	1. Have small group of faculty using modules at first, to demonstrate educational benefits 2. Schedule workshops to aid in change of role perception and to assist with learning about module development and use 3. Establish incentives for use of nontraditional approaches that increase learning effectiveness 4. Set up research projects that will demonstrate the value of individualized instruction 5. Establish mechanisms that maintain teacher contact with the student 6. Provide recognition for involvement in efforts to increase teaching effectiveness, such as that found with involvement in research, community service, and committee work 7. Provide release time for faculty to develop learning materials and evaluate their effectiveness
Difficulty in keeping modules updated and revised related to rapid proliferation of knowledge	1. Provide faculty release time for revision work 2. Structure modules so that resources used can be readily changed without altering the total package 3. Utilize available instructional design/evaluation personnel to help with process 4. Develop modules around major concepts rather than specific content, which changes rapidly
Lack of appropriate learning resources (software) related to cost and failure of commercial media to meet local needs	1. Provide time and budget for in-house development of learning materials 2. Write instructional grant proposals that will provide additional funding 3. Let media publishers know what is needed and work with them to develop materials 4. Collect data to establish need for support of budget requests 5. Adjust commercial media (within copyright limitations) to meet local needs (adding slides, printed materials, or audiotape)

intent here is to list potential problem areas and to identify possible interventions for dealing with them. Table 12-2 outlines three potential problems in relation to student role, whereas Table 12-3 identifies three potential problems in relation to teacher role and learning resources. Suggested interventions for dealing with each problem are given. Problems and interventions are examples only and are not presented as an exhaustive list.

SUMMARY

The use of the learning module as an instructional system for indi- vidualizing instruction has been discussed. The term learning module has been defined and a suggested system for developing modules given. Elements of learning modules were identified and discussed. Use of modules was described, including common uses and patterns for timing, sequencing, sociological format, and grading. Lasty, six potential prob- lems associated with modular learning in the areas of student role, teacher role, and availability of learning resources were identified, and several possible interventions related to each area were given.

APPENDIX 1: SAMPLE MODULE
FETAL CIRCULATION AND CHANGES AT BIRTH

Table of Contents

Introduction

An understanding of the anatomy and physiology of fetal circulation provides a basis for the study of congenital heart abnormalities and increases the ease with which one can learn about the specific abnormalities. If the content of this module is mastered, you will be well prepared to study those congenital heart abnormalities referred to as cardiac shunts.

Terminal Goal

Upon completion of this module, you will have a knowledge and understanding of the anatomy and physiology of fetal circulation and those changes that normally occur at the time of birth.

Directions

Proceed through the module as follows:

1. Read the section on prerequisites below and review as necessary.
2. Read the objectives for the module on page 182.
3. Take the pretest if you feel you have prior background or experience that prepares you to meet the objectives. Grade the pretest using the key provided at the end of the module.
4. If you score less than 100% on the pretest, use the resources listed on page 181 to complete those activities and self-checks that have to do with the objectives you did not reach. If you did score 100% on the pretest, you do not need to do further work on the module.
5. Complete the posttest. Repeat activities if necessary in order to reach the objectives. If the pretest has not been completed previously, you may also wish to use it to further validate your learning.

Prerequisites

It is essential that you have certain background knowledge about normal circulation before you can expect to complete this module successfully. Be sure you are able to complete the following before beginning to work on the module. If you need help to meet the prerequisites, a list of suggested resources is given.

1. Name the four chambers of the heart.
2. Name the two veins that return blood from the body to the right atrium.
3. Name the artery that takes blood from the right ventricle to the lungs.
4. Name the artery that takes blood from the left ventricle to the body.
5. Define the terms: oxygenated blood, deoxygenated blood, systemic circulation, pulmonary circulation, artery, vein, arterial blood, and venous blood.
6. State whether the blood found in each heart chamber and each major artery leaving the heart contains oxygenated or deoxygenated blood.

7. Trace the route of blood flow from the time it enters the right atrium until the time it leaves the heart via the aorta.

Sources for satisfying the prerequisites:

1. Any college or university level anatomy and physiology text.
2. Guyton, A.C. *Textbook of medical physiology* (5th ed.). Philadelphia: Saunders, 1976.
3. Ross Laboratories. The normal heart. (Chart available in NLRC.)

Learning Resources for Module

Use any of the resources listed below as directed in each of the activities. The choice is yours and depends on which you would prefer to use or have available.

1. Ross Laboratories. Fetal circulation (chart available in NLRC), or a labeled diagram of fetal circulation from any other reference.
2. Any recent medical, nursing, or anatomy and physiology text that includes content about fetal circulation. Suggested references:
   Jenscn, M.D., Benson, R.C., and Bobak, I.M. *Maternity care—the nurse and the family*. St. Louis: Mosby, 1977, pp. 117–119.
   Guyton, A.C. *Textbook of medical physiology* (5th ed.). Philadelphia: Saunders, 1976, pp. 1125–1127.
   Ross Laboratories. Fetal circulation. (Discussion sheet available in NLRC.)

Pretest

100% mastery required. Each question is keyed to the objective(s) that it relates to. Complete the activities and self-checks for any objective that you cannot meet.

1. Place the letter of the item in column B in the blank next to the item it best matches or explains in column A. All items in the second column will not be needed. (Objectives 1, 2, and 3)

A	B
____ 1. Umbilical vein	A. carries deoxygenated blood from the fetus to the placenta
____ 2. Umbilical arteries	B. an opening between the right and left atria
____ 3. Foramen ovale	C. an increased RBC count
____ 4. Ductus arteriosus	D. carries oxygenated blood from the placenta to the fetus
____ 5. Polycythemia	E. an increased WBC count
	F. an opening between the right and left ventricles
	G. a connection between the aorta and the pulmonary artery

2. State the normal number of each of the blood vessel types found in the umbilical cord. (Objective 1)

3. What is the purpose of the foramen ovale and the ductus arteriosus in fetal circulation? (Objective 2)

4. In fetal circulation, the systolic pressure is greatest on the _____ side of the heart; therefore, the direction of blood flow through the foramen ovale is toward the _____ atrium. (Objective 2)

5. The blood found in the aorta of the fetus is _____ (oxygenated, deoxygenated, or a mixture of the two). (Objective 4)

6. What is the purpose of polycythemia in fetal circulation? (Objective 3)

7. Describe the alteration in relation to the route of blood flow through the heart, the pulmonary artery, and the aorta that should occur at birth or shortly after birth. Include the closure of fetal structures, changes in direction of blood flow, and changes in pressure and oxygenation levels, if any, in the chambers and major vessels of the heart. (Use back of page or a separate sheet of paper.) (Objective 5)

8. Look at the two unlabeled charts depicting fetal circulation and normal circulation after birth. Identify which is which. (Objective 6)

Learning Objectives

Upon completion of the activities, you will be able to:

1. Name the two blood vessel types found in the umbilical cord, state the number of each, identify whether the blood found in each is oxygenated or deoxygenated, and state the direction of blood flow in each in relation to the fetus and the placenta.

2. Name and locate the two shunts that are normal in fetal circulation and state the purpose of each.

3. Define the term polycythemia, and state its purpose in fetal circulation.

4. Label a diagram of fetal circulation indicating differences in systolic pressure between the left and right side of the heart and between the aorta and pulmonary artery, the direction of blood flow through the foramen ovale and ductus arteriosus, and the level of oxygenation of blood in the four chambers of the heart and its four major vessels.

5. Describe the changes in circulation that should occur at birth or shortly after birth, including the closure of fetal structures, changes in direction of blood flow, and changes in pressure and oxygenation levels in the chambers and major vessels of the heart. Label a diagram indicating these changes.

6. Distinguish between two unlabeled diagrams or slides depicting fetal circulation and normal circulation after birth within the heart, pulmonary artery, and aorta.

Learning Activity 1 (Objectives 1, 2, and 3)

Refer to a labeled diagram of fetal circulation and a reference source that describes fetal circulation and answer the following questions:

1. What are the names of the blood vessels found in the umbilical cord?

2. How many of each of these vessels are there?

3. What is the direction of blood flow in each vessel in relation to the fetus?

4. Describe each vessel regarding content of oxygenated or deoxygenated blood.

5. What is the name of the fetal opening between the left atrium and the right atrium?

6. What is the name of the fetal structure connecting the pulmonary artery with the aorta?

7. What is the primary purpose of the two structures identified in questions 5 and 6?

8. Define the term polycythemia, and state its purpose in fetal circulation.

Activity 1 Self-Check

1. Name the vascular structures in the umbilical cord and state the number of each.

2. Place the letter of the item in column B in the blank next to the item it best matches or explains in column A. All items in the second column will not be needed.

A	B
____ 1. Umbilical vein	A. carries deoxygenated blood from the fetus to the placenta
____ 2. Umbilical arteries	B. an opening between the right and left atria
____ 3. Foramen ovale	C. an increased RBC count
____ 4. Ductus arteriosus	D. carries oxygenated blood from the placenta to the fetus
____ 5. Polycythemia	E. an increased WBC count
	F. an opening between the right and left ventricles
	G. a connection between the aorta and the pulmonary artery

3. On this diagram name and locate the two fetal structures that cause a normal shunting of blood before birth.

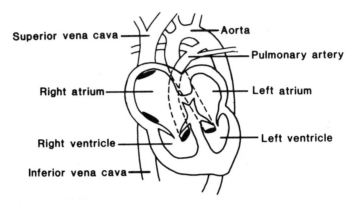

4. Write a sentence stating the primary purpose of the two structures identified in 3.
5. What function does polycythemia serve in fetal circulation?

Check your answers with those provided at the end of the module. If you did not answer all questions correctly, return to Activity 1, review the content, and repeat the Self-Check.

Learning Activity 2 (Objective 4)

Refer to any of the resources on fetal circulation and answer the following questions:

1. Where is the systolic pressure greater in fetal circulation? Right or left side of heart? Aorta or pulmonary artery?
2. What is the direction of the blood flow through the foramen ovale and the ductus arteriosus?
3. Determine the level of oxygenation of the blood in each of the following structures. Write "high" if highly oxygenated, "low" if deoxygenated, and "mix" if a mixture of oxygenated and deoxygenated blood.

　　_____ superior vena cava
　　_____ umbilical vein
　　_____ inferior vena cava
　　_____ left atrium and left ventricle
　　_____ right atrium
　　_____ right ventricle
　　_____ pulmonary artery
　　_____ aorta

Activity 2 Self-Check

Label the following diagram of the fetal heart according to the directions below.

1. Place an "X" on the side of the heart and on the artery that has the highest systolic pressure.
2. Indicate with an arrow the direction of blood flow through the foramen ovale and the ductus arteriosus.
3. Indicate the level of oxygenation of blood in each of the following: the superior vena cava, the inferior vena cava, the left atrium and ventricle, the right atrium, the right ventricle, the pulmonary artery, and the aorta. Write "high" or color in with a red marker if highly oxygenated. Write "low" or color in with a blue marker if deoxygenated. Write "mix" or color in with a green marker if a mixture of oxygenated and deoxygenated blood.

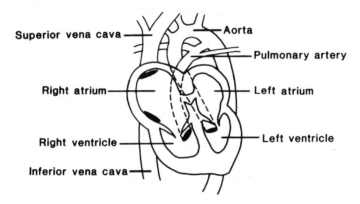

Check your completed diagram with the answers provided at the end of the module. If any answers were not correct, return to activity 2 for further study and then repeat the Self-Check.

Learning Activity 3 (Objective 5)

There are many physiological adjustments that the newborn baby must make. These adjustments are great in the first moments of life and the first few hours after birth. Their magnitude is illustrated by the fact that there is a high rate of mortality during the first 24 hours after birth with 30 percent of all infants who die in the first year of life dying during the first 24 hours.

Significant changes occur in the circulatory system at or shortly after birth. These changes involve both structural and functional aspects. Use any of the resources to write a description of the changes in the following areas:

1. Closure or obliteration of fetal structures. What are the structures, and why does each close?

2. With the closure of the structures, describe the change in the route of blood flow through the heart, the pulmonary artery, and the aorta.

3. With the closure of the structures, describe the change in the oxygenation level in the right side of the heart and pulmonary artery (pulmonary circulation), and the left side of the heart and the aorta (systemic circulation).

Activity 3 Self-Check

Label the following diagram of the fetal heart according to the directions below.

1. Place an "X" on the side of the heart and in the artery that have the highest systolic pressure after birth.

2. Draw a line to show which structures close at birth or shortly after birth.

3. Indicate level of oxygenation of blood in each of the following structures after birth: the superior vena cava, the inferior vena cava, the right atrium and ventricle, the pulmonary artery, the left atrium and ventricle, and the aorta. White "high" or color in with a red marker if highly oxygenated. Write "low" or color in with a blue marker if deoxygenated. Write "mix" or color in with a green marker if a mixture of oxygenated and deoxygenated blood.

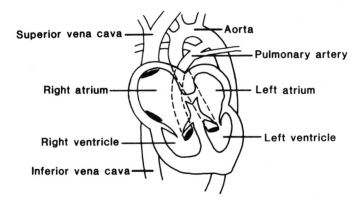

Check your completed diagram with the answers provided at the end of the module. If you missed any question, restudy Activity 3 and, then, repeat the Self-Check.

You have completed the learning activities for this module and may now proceed to the posttest, which begins below.

Posttest

100% mastery is required. If you miss any question or part of any question, review that section of the module until you can achieve 100% mastery. You may also wish to complete the pretest to further validate your learning.

1. What is the purpose of polycythemia in fetal circulation? (Objective 3)
2. What is the purpose of the ductus arteriosus? (Objective 2)
3. Place the letter of the item in column B in the blank next to the item it best matches or explains in column A. All items in the second column will not be used. (Objectives 1, 2, and 3)

A	B
____ 1. Umbilical vein	A. carries deoxygenated blood from the fetus to the placenta
____ 2. Umbilical arteries	B. an opening between the right and left atria
____ 3. Foramen ovale	C. an increased RBC count
____ 4. Ductus arteriosus	D. carries oxygenated blood from the placenta to the fetus
____ 5. Polycythemia	E. an increased WBC count
	F. an opening between the right and left ventricles
	G. a connection between the aorta and the pulmonary artery

4. Which two fetal blood vessels contain blood that is the most highly oxygenated? (Objectives 1 and 4)
5. In fetal circulation, systolic pressure is greater on the _____ side of the heart and in the _____ (pulmonary artery or aorta). (Objective 4)
6. In fetal circulation, the direction of blood flow through the ductus arteriosus is (Objectives 2 and 4)
   A. from the pulmonary artery to the aorta
   B. from the aorta to the pulmonary artery
   C. from the right atrium to the left atrium
   D. from the left atrium to the right atrium
7. In fetal circulation, there is a mixture of oxygenated and deoxygenated blood in the (Objective 4)
   A. right atrium
   B. pulmonary artery
   C. left ventricle
   D. descending aorta
   E. inferior vena cava
8. Indicate with an "X" in the blank if that situation normally exists in the newborn infant: (Objective 5)
   ____ A. a shunting of blood between the right and left atria
   ____ B. highly oxygenated blood in the aorta
   ____ C. an open ductus arteriosus
   ____ D. deoxygenated blood in the right atrium

9. After birth, systolic pressure is greater on the _____ side of the heart and in the _____ (pulmonary artery or aorta). (Objective 5)

10. What occurs at birth to alter the direction of blood flow and the level of oxygenation of blood in the aorta? (Objective 5)

11. After birth, the structure that contains the most highly oxygenated blood is the (Objective 5)
    A. right atrium
    B. pulmonary artery
    C. aorta
    D. inferior vena cava
    E. umbilical vein

12. Project the two slides of fetal circulation and normal circulation after birth on the screen. Distinguish between the two by identifying which is which. (Obtain slides in the NLRC.)

Keys to Pretest, Activity Self-Checks, and Posttest

PRETEST KEY

1. D, A, B, G, C.
2. One umbilical vein and two umbilical arteries.
3. To bypass the nonfunctioning fetal lungs in order to send blood, which is relatively high in oxygen, to body cells.
4. Right, left.
5. A mixture. Although a mixture, the blood in the aorta proximal to the ductus arteriosus is more highly oxygenated than that distal to this structure.
6. The body attempts to compensate for the resulting mixture of oxygenated and deoxygenated blood going into the systemic circulation by increasing RBC count and, thus, oxygen-carrying capacity.
7. The foramen ovale and ductus arteriosus should close, causing a cessation of shunting of blood from the right atrium to the left atrium and from the pulmonary artery to the aorta. A normal adult circulation pattern is begun. Pressure and oxygenation in systemic circulation are greater than that in pulmonary circulation.
8. Chart A is circulation after birth. Chart B is fetal circulation.

KEYS TO ACTIVITY SELF-CHECKS
Activity 1

1. Two umbilical arteries and one umbilical vein.
2. D, A, B, G, C.
3. Foramen ovale identified as opening between right and left atria; ductus arteriosus identified as connection between pulmonary artery and aorta.

4. These structures allow part of the more highly oxygenated blood to bypass the nonfunctioning fetal lungs and to send blood, which is relatively high in oxygen, to body cells.

5. The body attempts to compensate for the resulting mixtue of oxygenated and deoxygenated blood going into the systemic circulation by increasing RBC count and, thus, oxygen-carrying capacity.

Activity 2

1. "X" should be placed on the right side of heart and pulmonary artery.

2. Blood flows through foramen ovale from the right atrium into the left atrium and through the ductus arteriosus from the pulmonary artery into the aorta.

3. *Low* superior vena cava; *mix* inferior vena cava; *mix* right atrium (note: although both are passing through the right atrium, most of the deoxygenated blood from the superior vena cava is directed downward into the right ventricle, and most of the more highly oxygenated blood from the inferior vena cava is directed straight across through the foramen ovale into the left atrium); *mix* left atrium and left ventricle; *mix* pulmonary artery; *mix* aorta (note: although there is a mix, the blood in the aorta, which goes to the head and upper body, is more highly oxygenated than that in the aorta distal to the ductus arteriosus since additional deoxygenated blood is shunted into the aorta at that point.

Activity 3

1. "X" should be placed on the left side of the heart and on the aorta.

2. Lines should be drawn to close foramen ovale and ductus arteriosus.

3. *Low* superior vena cava, inferior vena cava, right atrium and ventricle, and pulmonary artery. *High* left atrium and ventricle, aorta. Should no longer be any mixture of the two in any structure.

POSTTEST KEY

1. To assure adequate oxygenation of body cells by increasing oxygen-carrying capacity by increasing number of RBC.

2. To allow blood to be diverted from the pulmonary artery into the aorta in order to bypass the nonfunctioning fetal lungs.

3. D, A, B, G, C.

4. The umbilical vein and the inferior vena cava.

5. *Right* side and in the *pulmonary artery*.

6. A.

7. A, B, C, D, and E. Although there is a mixture in all of these, there is a relatively high oxygenation of blood in the right atrium and, thus, in the left side of heart and aorta proximal to the ductus arteriosus.

8. "X" should be placed next to B and D.

9. *Left* side and in the *aorta*.

10. Fetal lungs begin to function, which decreases resistance to blood flow and, thus, reduces pressure on right side of heart and in the pulmonary artery. Loss of placental blood flow increases systemic pressure on the left side of the heart and in the aorta. These changes in pressure cause the foramen ovale to close. The flow of oxygenated blood through the ductus arteriosus causes it to become nonfunctional; it is later occluded by growth of fibrous tissue.

11. C.

12. Slide A is normal circulation after birth. Slide B is fetal circulation.

MODULE FEEDBACK FORM

Title of module: _____

1. Make a check and comment in each of following areas:

Area	Relevance		Clarity		Organization		Comments
	Yes	No	Yes	No	Yes	No	
a. Content							
b. Objectives							
c. Activities							
d. Media (including articles and AV)							
e. Pre- and posttests and check-points							

2. Directions to the student were (circle one)
   very clear   very unclear
     1   2   3   4   5
   comments:

3. List those things about the module that you liked.

4. List those things about the module that you did not like.

5. What was your overall impression of the module? (circle one)
   excellent   poor
     1   2   3   4   5
   comments:

6. Please made specific suggestion(s) for revision of the module. (Use back of form, if necessary.)

13

Using Learning Contracts

The contract as a formal legal agreement is well known in American society. It is usually written but can be verbal. It binds two or more people or agencies in an agreement to carry out specific behaviors, usually within a certain period of time. It is essential before signing the contract that all parties are in agreement about goals and have a clear understanding of responsibilities of each participant. Legal contracts are often renegotiated when the situation of either party alters the ability to meet commitments.

In traditional learning situations, the contract between the teacher and a student is usually implied rather than explicit. Both teacher and student have certain expectations of themselves and each other. The student expects the teacher to provide appropriate learning opportunities so that the student can learn what the teacher requires. At the same time, the teacher expects that students will be motivated to carry out assigned activities and work to their highest level of potential to try to achieve the desired learning outcomes. Each participant may have greater expectations of the other person than of themself, have unrealistic expectations, or feel betrayed when the other party does not behave as anticipated. The common results of such a situation are unclear expectations, unmet goals, and anxiety and frustration.

The type of contract referred to in this chapter is one in which there is an explicit agreement between the teacher and a student or group of students. It identifies exactly what each will do. It denotes a mutuality in establishing learning objectives, selecting resources and activities, and evaluating learning outcomes. It emphasizes learning rather than grading.

The use of learning contracts can be traced back to 1919 (Dewey, 1922). The method was first developed by Parkhurst in the use of "laboratory plans" made up of projects or units of study that were to be completed within a designated time period. Later, it was referred to as the Dalton Plan. More recently, attention has been given to variations in learning styles (Witkin, 1973; Witkin & Moore, 1974; Kagan & Kogan, 1970) and the needs of adult learners (Tough, 1981; Knowles, 1978).

In recent years the student population in basic programs of nursing education has become more and more varied and is made up of greater numbers of adult learners. Adults also comprise the learner group in continuing education programs, in-service education, and graduate programs in nursing. Recognizing this, the learning contract and other methods have been used in some settings in an effort to address differences among individuals and the needs of adult learners.

The philosophy behind the learning contract has been applied in nursing education to make up of deficiencies by marginal or failing students (Paduano, 1979); elective courses at the undergraduate level (Valadez & Heusinkveld, 1977); required courses at the undergraduate level (Bouchard & Steels, 1980; Crancer et al., 1977; Aavedal et al., 1975; Marriner, 1974; Layton, 1972; Rauen & Waring, 1972; Martens, 1981; M. DeMeneses, personal communication, April 21, 1981) and graduate level (M. DeMeneses, personal communication, April 21, 1981); and in-service or continuing education (Dougan, 1980; Reinhart, 1977; Smith, 1980).

In some higher education settings (Craig, 1975; Feeney & Riley, 1975; Worby, 1979) the learning contract is the only method used for the entire educational experience; however, traditional methods such as lectures, complete courses, and the like are often used as part of the contract.

DEFINITIONS

Learning contracts have been described by Berte (1975a), Lindquist (1975), Knowles (1978), and Clark (1981). Each presents a description of what a learning contract is from a particular perspective. Definitions of terms associated with contract learning as used in this chapter are given below.

LEARNING CONTRACT (LC):   An individualized learning plan that has been mutually negotiated and designed by a teacher (or committee) and a student (or
group of students).* Although not a legally binding document, it is a written,
signed agreement, which specifies the exact responsibilities of all parties in
helping the student achieve certain learning outcomes and the reward that is
forthcoming to the student once commitments have been met. It provides
opportunities for a student to learn independently at a self-determined rate
and includes a variety of learning resources/activities through which the student can obtain required information. It is usually established for a set period
of time, such as a semester or quarter; however, the time can be open-ended.
Depending on specific circumstances and limitations, it may be renegotiated or
modified at any time should unexpected contingencies arise or the student
desire to increase or decrease the amount or quality of work.

CONTRACTING: The process of teacher-student negotiation and interaction in
designing the final learning plan (the learning contract).

CONTRACT LEARNING: Applies to either the process of using LCs or the specific
learning gains associated with their use.

VALUES

Three fundamental principles underlie the use of LCs: (1) individuals
are different; (2) adults are self-directing; and (3) learning is a lifelong
process. Research by Witkin (1973), Witkin and Moore (1974), and Kagan and Kogan (1970) provide evidence of unique learning styles among
individuals. Others (Dunn & Dunn, 1978; Kolb, 1976) have analyzed
variations in learning styles through the development of instruments for
that purpose.

    There is widespread agreement about the capacity of LCs to indi-
vidualize instruction by responding to differences in learning needs,
styles, and interests (Boyd, 1979; Berte, 1975b; Rauen & Waring, 1972;
Worby, 1979; Valadez & Heusinkveld, 1977; Dash, 1970; Bouchard &
Steels, 1980). The LC allows individual differences in work rate by permitting those who want to progress more quickly to do so and allowing
those who require or desire more time, for whatever reason, to have it.
Individual styles and interests are recognized by the use of varied resources and activities or the provision of student options in types of

---

*Although the terms teacher and student are used throughout this chapter, they apply
equally to any situation in which mentor/learner relationships are established, such as that
of the staff development instructor-staff nurse.

resources and activities. Thus, the choices that are made can reflect personal interests and unique ways of learning, as well as greater relevancy to life and professional experiences and goals of the student.

It is clear, then, that by nature the LC is student-centered; however, that does not mean that the student is left totally alone. Rather, the teacher has a vital, although nontraditional, role in helping the student learn. However, in contrast to most traditional education, the main foci are learning rather than instruction and active rather than passive involvement of the learner. There is mutual understanding of the expectations of both teacher and student. The student participates in developing the LC and agrees to the standards for personal achievement; consequently, there is less need for competition with other students and less anxiety and frustration over grades.

LCs offer fulfillment of the adult's need to be self-directing. Tough (1971, 1981) and Knowles (1978) have established the ability of adult learners to design and complete their own learning projects. Knowles credits contract learning with being the single most effective tool for adult education. He says, "It solves the problem of the wide range of backgrounds, education, experience, interests, motivations, and abilities that characterize most adult groups by providing a way for individuals . . . to tailor-make their own learning plans" (Knowles, 1978, p. 127). The LC allows adult learners to build on broad human experiences and develop learning situations that help them to deal with problems they are facing in the real world. Through mutual planning and decision-making, the learner participates more fully and is more highly committed to the outcomes set by the LC. In research reported by Lehmann (1975), surveying adult learners in a setting that used LCs exclusively, the majority of those surveyed felt that they had gained in intellectual competence and sense of self-confidence and that contract learning was superior and more relevant than traditional education.

Many adults and other learners, however, have been conditioned through traditional educational practices to be dependent in the learning situation (Knowles, 1978). For them, the process of negotiating and carrying out the activities of a LC fosters the development of independence and self-direction (Reinhart, 1977; Lehmann, 1975). Since students are heavily involved in discussions about objectives, resources and activities, and ways of evaluating, they are forced to think about personal and educational goals and take personal responsibility for their own learning.

Increased independence and responsibility for learning also help to teach students that learning is a lifelong process over which they have control. Through the use of an LC students have the opportunity to learn how to learn (Chickering, 1975), a skill that is vital for continued learning after graduation. Students who learn to problem solve, manage their own learning, and develop independent, creative ways of thinking are better prepared to deal with the knowledge explosion and rapid changes associated with a field such as nursing.

ELEMENTS

Different authors have identified and described the various elements of the LC (Worby, 1979; Knowles, 1978; Paduano, 1979; Bouchard & Steels, 1980; Moran, 1980; Clark, 1981; Lehmann, 1975). Although the organization and relationships among the elements vary with individual and institutional practices, the following list is given as the framework for discussion in this chapter:

1. A general statement of the student's long range goals, purposes, and objectives.
2. Clear statements of the specific objectives/learning outcomes to be accomplished upon completion of the LC.
3. A description of the learning activities to be completed by the student and the learning resources to be used, including identification of responsibilities of the teacher or other mentor and anyone else who may be supervising the work of the student.
4. Identification of what is to be used as evidence that objectives have been met and the criteria by which the evidence will be evaluated. Any responsibilities of the teacher or other personnel are also identified.
5. An indication of what reward the student is to receive upon satisfactory completion of the LC.
6. Time frame to be used.
7. Signatures of the teacher (or other mentor) and student.

Each of the elements will be discussed briefly and an example given in a sample learning contract shown in Appendix 1 (page 207).

General Statement

The general statement of the student's long-range goals, purposes, and objectives is helpful in setting the parameters of the LC in relation to the specific objectives. For example, a student who wants to complete an LC in some area of pediatrics might have the general statement shown in the sample learning contract.

Specific Objectives

Objectives in an LC are usually identified by the student involved; however, once identified they are negotiated and refined in consultation with the teacher. A student often requires help in narrowing the objectives to realistic levels and in stating them so that they can be objectively evaluated. The teacher must make sure that the objectives are relevant to curricular goals, appropriate to the general goals of the student, and of satisfactory depth and breadth to warrant the reward established by the LC. See Appendix 1 for examples of objectives.

Learning Activities and Resources

The learning resources used in an LC should be available, up-to-date, and directly relevant to the desired learning outcomes. Depending on the subject matter and the availability of resources, various types should be used—reading, listening, viewing, and manipulating. The resources can include regular, correspondence or noncredit courses, workshops, textbooks and articles, audiovisual programs, models, travel, and people. Some resources may not be identified ahead of time but, rather, have the student locate additional learning resources as part of the LC.

In utilization of the resources, attention should be given to providing choices to the student. Certain activities can be required while the student selects another from a list of two or more. Activities can include such varied things as reading a textbook or article; viewing/listening to an audiovisual program; attending conferences, workshops, or scheduled classes; participating in field/practicum experiences; participating in study groups, committees, or task groups; visiting people or community agencies; doing an interview; completing research projects or surveys; conducting a library or computerized search; critiquing a chapter, article, or research report; or doing volunteer work. The extent of possibilities is only limited by one's imagination and creativity.

See the sample contract for examples of learning activities and resources. Note that responsibilities of the mentor and others are identified. The mentor may need to meet with the student at intervals for conferences to determine progress or provide help if needed. Appointments for the conferences can be scheduled or left to the responsibility of the student. The frequency varies with the type of contract, level of student, and extent of a student's self-direction and discipline. The highly motivated and self-disciplined student may require little help after the LC has been negotiated and knowledge of how to demonstrate accomplishment of the objectives is clear. The student who is less motivated or has difficulty in maintaining self-discipline will likely need more frequent conferences to verify understanding, check progress, and provide encouragement and praise.

Evidence of Accomplishment and Criteria of Evaluation

Tangible results of the activities and use of the resources must be identified. Evidence presented can include written reports, bibliography cards, logs, or journals; taped reports, logs, or journals; production of models or displays; development of mediated projects; development of care or teaching plans; oral reports to peers; preparation of an article for publication or filing in a resource center; and performance on attitudinal scales or standard tests, and in real or simulated situations. Again, the possibilities are limited only by the objectives of the LC and the imagination and creativity of the participants.

The student must be aware of how the evidence will be evaluated and what the options are if the evidence presented is determined to be unsatisfactory. Criteria for evaluation are vital in terms of credibility of the program, transfer of credit, and accreditation (Berte, 1975b). If the LC is being used for continuing education credit, a system must be established to validate accomplishments and award earned credit (Reinhart, 1977). The criteria for evaluation of each item must be shared with the student and/or mutually arrived at by the teacher and student. Either way, the student must be aware at the outset how the evaluation will be done. For example, if a care plan is used, a description of what must be included is identified. If an oral report is to be given, the student must know the length and how it will be evaluated. Often a rating scale is used for this purpose; if so, the student should have a copy to guide preparation of the report. The student's work may be evaluated by experts in the field, such as staff nurses working with a student in a clinical setting. The student, also, may participate in the evaluation process. Both Rogers (1951) and Tough (1971) consider self-evaluation to be an opportunity for growth and a legitimate form of assessment. Such an arrangement requires trust by the mentor since complete control over rewards and punishments is being relinquished (Boyd, 1979). See the sample LC for examples of evaluation measures and criteria. Note that different types of evaluation measures have been used and that the student is asked to complete an evaluation of the LC process and teacher, in addition to the self-evaluation.

Rewards

Satisfactory completion of the requirements of the LC leads to the student's receipt of some type of reward (besides the learning that has occurred). It may simply be credit for completion of an activity or project or it may involve the more formal granting of credit or a letter grade. In either case, the student must know what the options are should the evidence be judged as unsatisfactory. Will the student have an opportunity to do further work or to complete an alternate activity? Will the student who does not meet the LC receive a failing mark, an incomplete, a lower grade, or will additional time be allotted? See Appendix 1 for an example of the reward associated with the sample LC.

Time Frame

The student needs to know what time frame, if any, applies to the LC. If it involves total independence and self-direction, an open-ended time frame can be used. If time constraints exist, such as the end of a semester or quarter, the LC should include the required completion date. The projected completion date must take into account the time needed to evaluate the work that has been done and the possibility that additional work will be required. One way to decrease the need for additional work at the last minute is to set up a schedule of interim progress checks for presentation of portions of the evidence of accomplishment of objectives. Deadlines throughout the time of the LC can help to decrease procrastination (Boyd, 1979). If deadlines are found to be unrealistic or other problems arise, such as illness and unforeseen commitments, the contract can be renegotiated as long as the final completion date is met. Renegotiation, when necessary, is the responsibility of the student.

The time frame for the sample LC shown in Appendix 1 was 1 semester; however, it required 3 weeks to negotiate and finalize the LC and the completion date for presentation of evidence was 3 weeks before the end of the semester. What remained was approximately 10 weeks for the student to do the required work. An initial progress check was established and the student was given the option of presenting any other evidence at any time. For example, the care plan could be completed immediately after the clinical days and the exhibits could be done as part of either clinical day.

Signatures

The signatures required on all LCs are those of the mentor and the student. In addition, other signatures that may be required include those of people who are involved in some aspect of the LC. For example, a person who has agreed to supervise field work or evaluate the student's performance in some activity should formalize that agreement in some way. It may be by signing that section of the LC or it may be through a letter of agreement. Whatever the method used, the responsibilities and expectations of each person involved must be clearly spelled out and understood. Finally, all parties should receive a copy of the LC.

THE CONTRACTING PROCESS

The LC can be used with individuals or groups for one activity, a unit, or an entire course. It can be used for independent study, establishing expectations for certain grades, providing flexible programs for those with prior experience, or continuing education and professional growth.

One or more aspects of the process of using LCs have been discussed by different authors (Bouchard & Steels, 1980; Clark, 1981; Knowles, 1978; Aavedal et al., 1975; Cooper, 1980; Worby, 1979; Martens, 1981). Major areas of the process include orientation of the student, assessment of student needs, development of the plan, carrying out the required activities, and evaluation. Each of these will be discussed briefly.

Orientation

Since many students will not have used LCs before, orientation is vital. Significant areas to consider include the concepts and principles of self-directed learning and the components, purposes, and values of LCs. A handout summarizing major points and providing guidelines for LC development is useful. The orientation can take place in a group or individually, depending on the situation in which LCs are being used.

One portion of the orientation can be the completion of a mediated, independent study learning module in preparation for an initial group or individual orientation.

Students who have never had any real control over the learning situation may be suspicious at first. Those who have always been dependent in a learning situation may have difficulty in dealing with the increased responsibility and need for self-direction. Either will require ongoing assistance in order to alter previous notions about learning and develop the skills required in becoming a more active, independent learner.

Assessment of Needs

An important part of developing an LC is the assessment of individual needs and goals. Areas can include levels of competence, future professional goals, personal interests, and analysis of qualities, strengths, and limitations. The key question to be answered is, "What does the student want to learn and why?" The assessment can be completed during a one to-one conference between the teacher and student or the student can be asked to complete a self-assessment paper as part of the orientation process. In a well-developed LC program, the use of formal learning style inventories (as discussed in Chapter 11) will help students and teachers become aware of ways in which the students learn best and the variety of activities and resources that are needed. If used, the learning style inventory can be done during orientation so that the information gained is available to student and teacher at the time of an initial conference.

Development of the Plan

Once the actual plan is to be developed, energy is focused on how to go about achieving and evaluating learning objectives. As a basis for the initial teacher–student conference, in addition to the self-assessment, the student can be asked to complete a rough draft of ideas using an LC form. During the initial conference, such material is used to mutually establish roles and responsibilities, identify appropriate resources and activities, decide on evaluation procedures, agree on the amount of credit or other reward, and set time constraints, deadlines, and interim conferences. In most instances, the LC at this time is tentative; however, the student gains ideas and guidance about how to proceed. The student is then encouraged to continue the analysis of goals and objectives, find out what is available, and refine ideas for a later, scheduled meeting with the teacher for the final drafting of the LC. For students who have had no prior experience with LCs, it may be helpful to allow access to samples of completed LCs to help them gain ideas and increase understanding of the process.

An area that the teacher must personally consider is whether or not the necessary skills and expertise are available in one's self. If not, the teacher needs to help the student locate others who can provide the necessary service or refer the student to someone who is known to have the skills and expertise needed. In this way, the contracting process is one of learning for the teacher as well as the student. To have the student become aware of this adds to the knowledge that learning is a lifelong process.

Completing Required Activities

Once the LC has been established, the student proceeds to carry out activities that have been agreed upon by the teacher and student. The student should be encouraged to begin work immediately and develop, in areas where flexibility exists, a time frame in which to operate. Contact between the teacher and student should be maintained in some way so that the teacher is aware of progress and the student receives feedback and encouragement. It is desirable, especially for students who have never used an LC before or who have not developed self-discipline, to establish a schedule of conferences, either group or individual or both, during which there is assessment of progress, feedback and suggestions, and determination of any unexpected events and necessary changes.

Renegotiation is a key concept in the use of LCs. Students may not have a realistic view of capabilities or may become less (or more) motivated once involved in the LC. Thus, some students may overextend themselves beyond what is realistic, refocus their energies, or decide they can accomplish more (or less) than the contract states. In addition, unexpected events, including financial problems, family responsibilities, and illness, may interfere with the completion of the LC as planned. Negotiation can include an extension of time, a change of activities and resources, or a decrease or increase in the requirements with accompanying alteration in the amount of reward. If LCs are being used for letter grades, sharing the specific criteria for all grade levels with all students allows a student to "retreat" to a lower level or move up to a higher level, if desired.

Evaluation

Evaluation becomes an explicit part of the learning process when using LCs. It is clear to both teacher and student what the student must do to gain the rewards identified in the contract. Specific techniques depend on the unique design of the LC but can involve self-evaluation; teacher evaluation of performance, projects, or papers; evaluation by supervisors or preceptors; ratings by peers; and performance on tests. It is also helpful to have the student evaluate the LC process itself and the work of the teacher or other people involved in completion of the LC.

Faculty Roles

The faculty–student relationship implied in the contracting process is one of mutual trust, responsibility, and decision making. The use of LCs requires the development of new faculty roles and skills from those of traditional transmitter of information. In discussions of faculty roles (Cooper, 1980; Moran, 1980; Clark, 1981; Bradley, 1975; Dougan, 1980; Worby, 1979; Boyd, 1979), four primary categories related to the direct teacher–student relationship emerge: counselor/adviser, negotiator, facilitator, and evaluator. Each will be described briefly.

Counselor/Adviser. As a counselor/adviser, the faculty member helps the student to clarify professional and personal goals, understand general educational requirements, understand LC procedures and requirements, and establish a learning plan that is compatible with other areas of the student's life. Once the LC is established, the teacher helps the student to set priorities, contact other people who will be involved, and arrange the necessary experiences to achieve learning objectives.

Negotiator. As negotiator, the faculty member works with the student to establish the specific requirements of the LC. This requires a cooperative rather than adversary relationship and the ability to listen and question in a way that will move the student toward identification of personal learning goals and methods. The teacher can help the student become aware of reasonable requirements for the reward desired and establish evaluation methods and criteria that are relevant. Should contract disputes arise, either in initial or renegotiation processes, a mechanism for dealing with them should be available. If faculty and students know that there is a special committee or group of outside examiners who will be available to objectively review any disagreements, both will experience a greater sense of security.

Facilitator.   As facilitator, the faculty member is involved in the intellectual development of the student. The primary responsibility is to help students learn how to learn on their own. In this capacity, the teacher needs a knowledge of the variety of resources available or the ability to direct the student to other places to obtain desired information. Teachers should be aware of, and readily admit, any personal limitations and be ready to refer the student to others who are experts in particular areas. As facilitator, the teacher assists in arranging placements in community/clinical settings and is the liaison with them for receipt of reports about student performance or evaluations of the LC experience.

Evaluator.   As evaluator, the faculty member is involved in formative and summative evaluation of the student and the learning process. The teacher needs to provide the student with honest, regular, constructive criticism in a way that will motivate the student toward achievement of learning objectives. Once the LC is completed, the teacher either provides or obtains final evaluation of the products of achievement established by the contract.

RELATED APPLICATIONS

Although the discussion in this chapter centers on the use of LCs with individuals, they can also be used with groups of students (Bouchard & Steels, 1980). Group contracts are beneficial in bringing together diverse perspectives, values, and experiences and providing psychological support, criticism, and evaluation of one another's work (Clark, 1981). With group LCs, each member of the group must be held accountable for providing individual evidence of performance, particularly if each member is to receive an individual grade. If a group grade is to be given, it becomes the responsibility of the members of the group to see that all individuals contribute equally to the achievement of the LC.

The philosophy behind LCs can also be applied to other uses in nursing education and practice besides those directly associated with individual or group learning. Some possibilities include:

1. Development of student–nurse and patient–family contracts to en-

hance mutual goal-setting, understanding of expectations, responsibility, and accountability (Gustafson, 1977; Coombe et al., 1981; Sheridan & Smith, 1975; Aavedal et al., 1975; Sloan & Schommer, 1975; Langford, 1978)

2. Development of student–agency contracts to increase student commitment and accountability (Rose et al., 1978)
3. Development of self-contracts for personal and professional growth (Wilson & Tosti, 1972)

POTENTIAL FACULTY PROBLEMS

Several problems that may be encountered with students at each phase of the contracting process have been discussed earlier in this chapter. Three that are specific to faculty are mentioned here: teacher workload, faculty roles, and returns on efforts.

Teacher Workload

There is agreement that the workload of the teacher using LCs is potentially greater than with traditional education methods (Berte, 1975b; Bradley, 1975; Clark, 1981; McKeachie, 1978). Without question, teachers need a broad range of competencies to provide the individualized guidance required. New programs require significant planning and organizational efforts. The one-to-one contacts with students are frequent, especially in the early stages of contract negotiation. Some students who have had no prior experience with LCs or have difficulty with becoming self-directive may require continuing frequent contacts with the teacher. The investigation and development of outside resources is time-consuming, especially when the use of LCs is first started. The amount of paperwork and the precise number of evaluative measures exceed most traditional courses. Even when the actual time spent overall is not greater, it may seem that way since it is more continually demanding of the energies and attention of the teacher.

In dealing with the problem of possible faculty overload, McKeachie (1978) suggests that close attention be paid to the faculty side of the LC so that an excessive amount of one-to-one teaching time is avoided. Clark (1981) points out the importance of training programs to help faculty develop necessary skills and the desirability of decreasing other faculty commitments when a new course using LCs is initiated. Faculty overload can also be prevented by the provision of adequate secretarial, administrative, and instructional development support staff so that the teacher can concentrate on the actual teaching-learning process.

Faculty Roles

Faculty members who have had experience in traditional roles only and are comfortable in them may find it difficult to adopt new roles or become anxious when placed in situations requiring different ways of behaving. Some will continue to "lecture" in spite of the situation. Some resist relinquishing control over students in order to keep them in dependent roles. Many will feel threatened by the need to admit to students that their knowledge is limited in some areas.

It is vital, if individualized programs are to be successful, that faculty roles be redefined and special training programs used to help those already in teaching develop the awareness and skills associated with the use of LCs (Berte, 1975b). New programs have a greater chance for success if the faculty members associated with them are interested in providing instruction that is more individualized. Groups of faculty should be selected who are able to work well together and provide mutual support and education.

Those in teacher-training programs should be exposed to a variety of teaching-learning methods so that they will be more likely to use them later when they work with students. It is helpful for them to experience the method that they, in turn, can use as future instructors (M. DeMeneses, personal communication, April 21, 1981).

Returns on Efforts

As with other individualized strategies, the teacher who uses LCs may receive little, if any, positive feedback from peers and administrators. This is most likely to occur when the precise statements of expectations in LCs are viewed as "spoonfeeding," when efforts impact at the local level only, or when grades of students using LCs are higher than those of groups learning by traditional methods.

In dealing with this problem, the teacher using LCs will often have to educate peers and administrators about the reasonableness of increased grades when students are more aware of exactly what is expected. On the other hand, the teacher should make sure that the quality of work is adequate to merit the grade for which contracted. In line with this, grade level differentiation should be based on quality as well as quantity of work (McKeachie, 1978). Higher education settings also need to develop reward systems that recognize innovative teaching efforts at the same level as other professional accomplishments (Berte, 1975b). Ways in which teachers might help to hasten that occurrence include combining their use of innovative strategies with some type of research or sharing their experiences through publications and conferences.

SUMMARY

The LC provides a mechanism for individualizing instruction with individuals and groups and establishing a pattern of self-direction and lifelong learning. It can be used in a variety of situations for individual activities and units or entire courses. Certain elements must be included to provide clear direction to both teacher and student about expectations and how the learning will be evaluated. The contracting process involves orientation, assessment, planning, implementation, and evaluation. Negotiation and renegotiation can occur throughout the process. Certain faculty roles are required when LCs are used, several of them different from those in traditional education. As with other strategies, LCs have potential problems associated with both students and faculty. A few ideas for preventing or dealing with the problem areas are offered.

APPENDIX 1
SAMPLE LEARNING CONTRACT

Student Name:	Mentor Name:
Address:	Address:
Telephone:	Telephone:

Long-Range Goals, Purposes, and Objectives

My goal is to complete the requirements of a baccalaureate degree in nursing and to obtain employment in an acute care pediatric setting.

Specific Objectives

1. To engage in a comprehensive study of the use of play with hospitalized children.
2. To integrate this study with the care of a child in each of the following age groups: infant, toddler, preschooler, and school age.
3. To describe and analyze the effects of the use of play with children in each age group.
4. To gain greater understanding of the effects of illness and separation on young children.

Learning Activities and Resources

1. Select any text (less than 5 years old) on the nursing care of infants and children and (a) review the content related to growth and development of each age group and (b) read the material about the reactions of children of each age group to illness and separation. Prepare notes for each of the two areas in relation to each age group.
2. Contact the campus audiovisual center and arrange to view the film, "Let's Play Hospital." Take notes and write a brief reaction to the film in relation to each of the four objectives.
3. Contact the recreational therapist at the University Hospital and make arrangements to observe in that setting for at least a 4-hour period and to interview the therapist for approximately 30 minutes. The teacher will make a phone call to initiate the contact.
4. Schedule 2 clinical days of 8 hours each in the pediatric unit at Valley Hospital when an instructor is present. Arrange the time desired at least 2 weeks in advance with either M. Thompson or T. Taylor.
5. Read at least three journal articles or chapters specifically related to the use of play with hospitalized children and write a one-page reaction paper on each. Chapters must be in addition to those read in Activity 1. Articles and chapters can be either personally chosen or selected from a list obtained from M. Thompson.
6. Meet with M. Thompson on 2/23/82 at 10 a.m. to discuss progress and any problems. Present a plan for completing activities not finished before that date.

Evaluation

1. Prepare a written paper of not more than 10 double-spaced pages in which an integration of the theoretical study of the use of play with hospitalized children from the various resources is demonstrated.
2. Prepare a one-page care plan focusing on the use of play with one child in each age group. The care plan must include an identification of a specific

problem, a theoretical explanation of the problem, identification of at least two nursing approaches for dealing with the problem, an explanation of the rationale for selection of the approach, and the identification of at least two objective criteria for the evaluation of success of each approach.

3. Develop some type of model or game for use with each of the four different age groups. These will be demonstrated to the nurses working in the pediatric unit at Valley Hospital, and a brief theoretical explanation will be given for each. The demonstrations can take place during one of the two clinical days. The nurses will evaluate each demonstration in relation to its creativity, ease of use, and appropriateness to the age for which developed.

4. Upon completion of the LC, write an evaluation of the project in relation to achievement of objectives, and complete a teacher and self-evaluation using the rating forms provided.

Beginning date: 2/17/82   Ending date: 4/27/82

Credit: 1 unit of independent study under N180 to be used as an elective toward the degree

---

Student signature_____   Date _____

Mentor signature _____   Date _____

14

Using Computers
to Aid Learning

There is no doubt that computer technology is having a significant influence on many areas of our lives. Most readers are probably familiar with the everyday role of computers in automated banking, supermarket checkout, airline reservations, screening of income tax returns, and production of bank statements, billings, and junk mail. Applications that are common, although less apparent, include those in telephone and defense systems, medical diagnosis, air traffic control, assembly lines, weather forecasting, and predictions of business and political trends. Other applications, such as home management, financial planning, health record maintenance, and electronic mailing and newspapers, are now possible and may be commonplace in the near future.

Colleges and universities will soon be receiving students who are children of such technological trends. They will have been exposed to computers in every aspect of their lives—entertainment, daily living, and education. They will need computer skills for success in many professions. If students enter higher education in a field in which computers are not used for instruction, it may interfere with the student's ability to deal with massive amounts of information and technological changes, contribute to the culture shock of the computer illiterate, and impede success in work. In fact, Pipes (1980) predicts that those who are computer illiterate will, in the near future, be as helpless as those who are now unable to read and write. Because of the pervasive influence of computers, it is vital that each individual learn about the nature and applications of this powerful tool in order to gain full benefit from its potential and deal effectively with its power.

Computers have been used for several years on college and university campuses—for some things. Common uses include scheduling of classrooms and students, figuring payrolls, grading examinations, and providing statistical analyses of examination results and research data. In a few areas, computers have been used for instruction; however, this has centered primarily around learning *about* the computer rather than learning *with* the computer. It is clear that higher education has not made full use of the technology that is currently available. Whether or not computers become a common part of the educational scene in colleges and universities is dependent on a number of factors. (A few of the barriers will be discussed later in the chapter.) The Carnegie Commission Report on Higher Education (1972, p. 1) predicts that by the year 2,000, "a significant portion of instruction in higher education on campus may be carried on through informational technology. . . ." In light of current technological capabilities, that prediction could become a reality sooner than 2,000 and be broadened to include all arenas in which education can occur.

Certainly computers should not be used for everything, anymore than lectures should be used for everything. Only in variety can different types of content be effectively transmitted and needs of each student met. The task is to determine what portions of the educational process can best be handled by the computer and what is best done by the teacher. Once this is recognized, the activities of each should complement rather than compete with one another. When properly used, the computer can enhance the work of the instructor, provide greater individualization of learning, and increase flexibility of the learning process (Rockart & Morton, 1975).

The aim of this chapter is to provide nursing educators who have no prior computer experience with an overview of how the computer can be used to facilitate teaching and learning. The primary focus is on those educational functions involving direct interaction between a student and a computer. It is not concerned with such topics as computer programming or the intricacies of computer operations. The reader is referred to references given for technical and more indepth information.

DEFINITIONS

A few basic definitions of computer terminology are given below. An effort has been made to state them in nontechnical language, while at the same time introducing a few common computer terms. The definitions are given in what seems to be a logical and sequential, rather than alphabetical, order.

COMPUTER: That part of the computer system in which data storage and manipulation occur and in which the operations of the system are controlled (Covvey & McAlister, 1980). A computer is referred to as the central processing unit (CPU). Currently, the major types are large (maxicomputer), medium (minicomputer), and small (microcomputer) in reference to size, computing power, and price. The present trend is toward increased miniaturization, greater capabilities, and lower prices.

TERMINAL: The device used to interact with a computer, that is, put information into a computer and/or receive information from a computer (Covvey & McAlister, 1980). It is often referred to as a peripheral unit and is made up of a keyboard similar to a typewriter and/or a televisionlike display screen called a cathode ray tube (CRT). The user converses with the computer by typing messages on the keyboard or using a "light pen" to indicate a desired response on the CRT. The computer responds by producing messages on the printer or displaying them on the CRT.

COMPUTER HARDWARE: The physical and electronic equipment of a computer system. Basic units include the computer (CPU) and the terminal.

INTELLIGENT TERMINAL: The term used to describe a terminal that has independent computing power in addition to being the interactive device between a user and the computer.

DUMB TERMINAL: A terminal that is used strictly as a communication device and does not possess any independent computing power (Covvey & McAlister, 1980).

COMPUTER PROGRAM: The set of instructions that directs the operation of a computer. Programs are usually contained on magnetic tape or disks similar to phonograph records.

COMPUTER SOFTWARE: The programs that tell the computer what to do in performing specific functions (Covvey & McAlister, 1980). Instructional programs are often called "courseware" (Rockart & Morton, 1975).

COMPUTER LANGUAGE: The alphabetical and numerical symbols required to communicate with a computer and develop a program. Examples are BASIC, FORTRAN, PILOT, and TUTOR, each with its unique applications and restrictions.

ON-LINE: A situation in which a user communicates directly with a computer (Covvey & McAlister, 1980) and in which there is immediate computer response to user input.

TIME-SHARING: A situation in which one computer serves many users, all on-line at the same time (Covvey & McAlister, 1980).

COMPUTER-BASED EDUCATION OR COMPUTER-BASED INSTRUCTION: A general term that encompasses the full range of uses of the computer in any part of the educational process (Hunter et al., 1975). Common subcategories are computer-assisted instruction and computer-managed instruction.

COMPUTER-ASSISTED (OR AIDED) INSTRUCTION (CAI):   Teaching and/or learning activities that use a computer as the main vehicle of delivery of content in a one-to-one interaction with a student. Common categories of CAI are tutorial, drill-and-practice, dialogue, inquiry, simulation, and gaming.

COMPUTER-MANAGED INSTRUCTION (CMI):   The use of a computer for instructional/teaching support functions, such as testing, record-keeping, monitoring of progress, diagnosis, and prescription (Milner, 1980).

COMPUTER NETWORK: A group of computer systems, the members of which can communicate with one another (Covvey & McAlister, 1980).

COMPUTER-ASSISTED INSTRUCTION

Computer-assisted instruction (CAI) involves the direct interaction between a student and a computer for the achievement of some learning task. Although some comments will be made about the management functions of computers (CMI), the remainder of this chapter will focus primarily on CAI. The areas of discussion are the general interactive process, types of CAI, research about effectiveness, values, extent of use and barriers to adoption, examples of application in nursing education, and future possibilities.

The General Interactive Process of CAI

Imagine a computer that contains a program designed to teach a student about a particular topic. Then imagine a student seated at a station or carrel containing a computer terminal. The computer and terminal may be in close proximity to one another or they may be located some distance apart with the communication link provided by telephone lines or a communication satellite. With a computer in which numerous programs are stored, different students can be using different programs at the same time. However, since the computer can process data and respond to the student so quickly, each student has the impression that the computer is interacting solely with that student.

The basic pattern of interaction is that the student signs on with the computer by typing specific information, such as name or code word, which the computer has been programmed to recognize. If visual display is available in the terminal, the messages typed by the student appear visually on the screen as they are typed. Once the student signs on and the computer welcomes the student, a selection of the desired program is made and the lesson begins. In some cases the student can send messages to the computer by touching a special sensor pen to an appropriate area on the display screen. In the future, computers may be developed that will be able to respond to a student's voice commands. Regardless of the method of input, the computer responds to each student message according to the directions in the stored instructional program. The specific pattern of interaction depends on the type of instructional program being used, for example, drill-and-practice. Messages from the computer to the student can be typewritten but they are more often displayed on the screen. Kinds of materials displayed include numbers (problems, numerical data); text (instructions, descriptions of clinical situations, information requested by the student, questions, feedback and messages of encouragement); and graphics (diagrams, charts, cardiograms). Auxiliary media—slides, videotape, audiocassette, microfiche—can be incorporated into the instructional program to provide variety of stimuli or allow student options. If the necessary hardware is available, these media are coordinated and controlled by the computer and presented at the terminal. If not, the student is directed by the computer to use the media located in the same station or carrel or to go to another location that has been designated for presentation of the media. Other supportive materials that provide a low-cost way of enhancing CAI without the need for expensive auxiliary equipment include visual materials (photographs, diagrams, charts); print materials (texts, articles, study guides); and anatomical models.

Throughout the process, the computer keeps track of student performance and provides that information to the teacher or student on demand. In response to student performance, the computer may branch to previous or new material, generate a personally-designed assignment, or tell the student to consult with the instructor.

Types of CAI

The basic types of CAI include tutorial, drill-and-practice, dialogue, inquiry, simulation, and gaming. All are interactive in the sense that the student communicates at a terminal with the author of the instructional program stored in the computer; however, the "human" quality of that interaction varies from a very simple question and answer format to a more complex form of open, free "conversation" as would occur in an actual teacher–student encounter. All require active participation by the student since the student is being continually asked to respond to questions, solve a problem, or make a decision. The instructional sequence of some are primarily program or author controlled while others are learner controlled; all, however, allow the student to control the pace at which study occurs.

Descriptions of the types of CAI are often confusing and overlapping. Although the term "tutorial" could be applied to any situation in which a computer is used in a teaching mode, it is generally given as one of the categories of CAI. Furthermore, it is possible for a single program to incorporate more than one type, leading to some of the confusion regarding specific characteristics of "pure" types. The aim here is to present each type in its "pure" form as interpreted from the use of a variety of references.

Several references were particularly useful in the preparation of this section (Farquhar et al., 1978; Holland & Hawkins, 1972; Hunter et al., 1975; Meadows, 1977; Rockart & Morton, 1975; and Zemper, 1978). These references present a much more extensive discussion of CAI, including examples from various fields, and the reader is referred to them for greater depth. Six types of CAI are identified and discussed. Table 14-6 is presented to summarize major points about each type.

Tutorial.   In the tutorial mode of CAI, it is the function of the computer to present new information to the student. In its simplest form, the content is presented in a linear series of factual statements interspersed with predetermined questions and responses from the computer. Typically the computer will present a content statement or question to which the student will respond, and, then, the computer will analyze and evaluate that response before deciding what material to present next. Rather than straight presentation of content, the computer can also be programmed to provide coaching to students in discovering new information and concepts for themselves.

In a more complex form, parallel sequences at different levels of difficulty can be available or the program can branch to bypass familiar material or to provide supplementary and remedial work before returning to the main instructional sequence. Most tutorial programs follow a basic programmed instruction technique; however, much more sophisticated branching is possible with the use of the computer. In addition, the computer program can provide corrective feedback, recommend activities for remediation of important background knowledge, or refer a student to the teacher for personal assistance in problematic areas. At any rate, the sequence of instruction is predetermined and controlled by the program with the student having no direct impact on the sequence or level of material that is presented. Its major advantage is that students are more aware of how well they are learning since the computer can analyze comprehension throughout the program and provide additional material based on that comprehension. In addition, the student has a high degree of control over the pacing and time at which study will take place. Table 14-1 is a sample program in the tutorial mode. The large type represents computer statements and response while student responses are in lower case.

Drill-and-Practice. In drill-and-practice the computer presents a series of questions or problems about material that has been previously learned, either by use of the computer or some other technique. Typically, the student is asked to make simple responses, such as filling in blanks, choosing from a list of alternatives, supplying a missing phrase, or providing the answer to a mathematical problem. Material that is well suited to a program of drill-and-practice includes simple, factual information requiring rote learning (e.g., medical terminology, abbreviations, and definitions) and the practice of computation skills (e.g., calculation of drug doses, body fluid needs, and caloric intake). A program of this type gives the student repeated opportunities for using the material or skills in relation to a given concept, thus helping to embed that concept in the student's knowledge base. It is possible to adjust the level of complexity of problems and questions based on individual student performance, thus the practice provided is at a level appropriate to each student. Depending on performance, some students may advance quickly while others who need it can be provided with repetitious practice or routed to necessary remedial work before returning to the drill-and-practice program. In this sense, and since the student has control over pacing and time of study, a drill-and-practice program is individualized. However, the control of sequence and level lies with the program rather than with the student. Table 14-2 presents an example from a program in the drill-and-practice mode.

Dialogue. Although the basic format for student–computer interaction is the same as with tutorial and drill-and-practice, with the dialogue mode that interaction takes on a more human, conversational quality in helping the student arrive at conclusions. A student's question, comment, or request for information initiates several possible responses from the computer—asking a question, coaching to try another approach, or guidance in reviewing previous material—much like that which occurs in an actual student–teacher encounter. As is the case in a direct teacher–student interaction, the conversation can move in differ-

Table 14-1

Excerpt from a Computer-Assisted Instruction Program Using the Tutorial Mode

```
HELLO!  I HAVE SOME INFORMATION TO GIVE YOU ABOUT
CALCULATION OF INTRAVENOUS (IV) FLUID RATES.
PLEASE TYPE IN YOUR FIRST NAME AND THEN HIT THE
"RETURN" KEY WHEN YOU ARE READY TO CONTINUE.

mary

FINE, MARY.  LET ME BEGIN BY TELLING YOU THAT YOU
NEED TO HAVE BASIC MATH SKILLS AND THE ABILITY TO
SOLVE A MATHEMATICAL PROBLEM ONCE NUMERICAL VALUES
HAVE BEEN PLACED INTO A FORMULA IN ORDER TO BE
SUCCESSFUL WITH THIS PROGRAM.  NEXT, YOU NEED TO
KNOW THAT VARIOUS IV SETS HAVE VARIOUS DROP
FACTORS--THAT IS, HOW MANY DROPS THAT SET DELIVERS
FOR EACH ML. OF SOLUTION.  THE INFORMATION ABOUT
DROP FACTOR IS OBTAINED BY READING THE PACKAGE
THAT THE IV SET COMES IN.  FOR EXAMPLE, VARIOUS
ADULT IV SETS DELIVER 10, 15, OR 20 GTTS. PER ML.
DEPENDING ON THE MANUFACTURER OF THE SET WHILE
PEDIATRIC IV SETS USUALLY DELIVER 60 GTTS. PER ML.

YOU MAY WANT TO STUDY THE ABOVE EXPLANATION BEFORE
PROCEEDING.  HIT THE "RETURN" KEY WHEN YOU ARE
READY TO GO ON.

ALL RIGHT, MARY, LET'S LOOK AT THE FIRST FORMULA
FOR SOLVING IV RATE PROBLEMS.  FLOW RATE IS
EXPRESSED AS VOLUME OF FLUID TO BE DELIVERED PER
UNIT OF TIME, USUALLY ML. PER HR. OR GTTS. PER
MIN.  FIRST, YOU NEED TO DETERMINE HOW MUCH FLUID
IS TO BE GIVEN IN 1 HR.  SOMETIMES, THE DOCTOR'S
ORDER IS WRITTEN THAT WAY--GIVE 125 ML. PER HR. OF
5% DEXTROSE IN WATER.  HOWEVER, GENERALLY WITH THE
ADULT PATIENT, THE ORDER WILL READ: GIVE 1000 ML.
5% DEXTROSE IN WATER IN 8 HRS. AND THE NURSE WILL
NEED TO DETERMINE THE HOURLY RATE.  THIS IS DONE
BY DIVIDING THE TOTAL VOLUME OF FLUID TO BE
INFUSED (IN ML.) BY THE INFUSION TIME (IN HRS.).
WITH THE LATTER EXAMPLE, THEN, ONE CAN DETERMINE
THAT 1000 ML. DIVIDED BY 8 HRS. EQUALS 125 ML. PER
HR.

YOU MAY WANT TO STUDY THE ABOVE EXPLANATION BEFORE
PROCEEDING.  HIT THE "RETURN" KEY WHEN YOU ARE
READY TO CONTINUE.

LET'S SEE IF YOU HAVE LEARNED THE MATERIAL JUST
PRESENTED BY HAVING YOU DO A PROBLEM SIMILAR TO
THAT IN THE EXAMPLE.  IF THE DOCTOR'S ORDER READS:
```

```
GIVE 1000 ML. 5% DEXTROSE IN WATER IN 6 HRS., WHAT
WILL BE THE AMOUNT TO BE ADMINISTERED EACH HR.?
TYPE YOUR ANSWER WHEN YOU ARE READY.
167 ml.
VERY GOOD, MARY.  1000 ML. DIVIDED BY 6 HRS.
EQUALS 166.6, ROUNDED TO 167 ML.  LET'S GO TO THE
NEXT STEP BY CALCULATING GTTS. PER MIN.  TO DO
THIS, YOU MUST DIVIDE THE VOLUME OF FLUID ORDERED
(IN ML.) BY THE LENGTH OF TIME IT IS TO INFUSE
(IN MIN.) AND MULTIPLY BY THE DROP FACTOR OF THE
IV SET.  THUS, THE FORMULA IS
```
$$\frac{\text{TOTAL VOLUME OF FLUID ORDERED (IN ML.)}}{\text{LENGTH OF TIME IT IS TO INFUSE (IN MIN.)}}$$
$$\text{X DROP FACTOR OF IV SET}$$
```
THUS, WITH THE PROBLEM YOU JUST CALCULATED (OF 167
ML. PER HR.) THE FORMULA WOULD BE FILLED IN AS
FOLLOWS WITH AN IV SET THAT DELIVERS 15 GTTS. PER
ML.
```
$$\frac{167}{60} \text{ X } 15 = 41.7 \text{ or } 42 \text{ GTTS. PER MIN.}$$

ent directions depending on student responses. The student is, thus, encouraged to explore and discover new learning. At any time, the student can ask for additional information or consult books, journals, other students, the teacher, or other experts in the field being studied.

Since the interaction is less structured and the uniqueness of an individual student's response can be addressed, the control of the learning sequence shifts from the computer program to the student. In order to provide such flexibility, however, it is necessary that the subject being studied be analyzed extensively to determine the different types of student questions and responses that are possible so that they may be incorporated into the program. A dialogue program is, therefore, more time-consuming and difficult to prepare.

Dialogue-type learning assistance with a computer has been used successfully by medical schools for teaching medical diagnosis. A variety of patient cases are stored in a computer, and the student interacts with the system as if dealing with a real patient. The computer program is designed to provide patient responses to questions, results of laboratory tests, changes in patient status, and so forth, that would normally be

Table 14-2

Excerpt from a Computer-Assisted Program Using Drill-and-Practice

```
PROBLEM 1.

    HOW MANY GRAMS OF GLUCOSE ARE THERE IN 1000
    ML. OF A 5% GLUCOSE SOLUTION?

    PLEASE TYPE YOUR ANSWER.

    5

    THE ANSWER GIVEN IS INCORRECT.   (HINT) DID YOU
    GIVE YOUR ANSWER IN RELATION TO 1000 ML.?
    LOOK AT THE PROBLEM AND TRY AGAIN.   PLEASE
    TYPE YOUR ANSWER.

    50

    THAT IS CORRECT.   1000 ML. X 0.05 (5% = 0.05)
    = 50 GRAMS.

PROBLEM 2.

    SINCE YOU HAD SOME TROUBLE WITH PROBLEM 1,
    LET'S HAVE YOU TRY ANOTHER ONE OF THE SAME
    TYPE.

    HOW MANY GRAMS OF GLUCOSE ARE THERE IN 250 ML.
    OF A 10% GLUCOSE SOLUTION?

    PLEASE TYPE YOUR ANSWER.

    25

    GOOD.   THE ANSWER IS CORRECT.   250 ML. X 0.10
    (10% = 0.10) = 25 GRAMS.
```

available upon request in an actual setting. The situation evolves much as it would in a real clinical setting as a result of student inquiries, diagnostic test results, treatments and interventions carried out. Throughout the process each student response or action is countered by suggestions, encouragement, or criticisms by the teacher through the program, which is similar to a real clinical teaching situation. In fact, dialogue-based computer situations are closely related to simulation and make up one of the major techniques of computer simulation of clinical encounters. (See Table 14-4 for an example from a program in the dialogue mode as part of a clinical problem-solving simulation activity.)

Inquiry. The inquiry mode is being utilized whenever the student has an opportunity to ask questions or request data from a computer program. Rather than guiding the student to correct answers or conclusions, as found in the drill-and-practice and tutorial modes, a program in the inquiry mode simply provides specific data requested or answers questions asked by the student. Thus, the student controls what information the computer presents by the type of inquiry made. No information is provided unless specifically requested by the student.

The inquiry aspect can be incorporated into any program using one or more types of CAI. The use of inquiry is particularly appropriate when numerical or clinical data is to be manipulated for the purpose of demonstrating either typical or unusual patterns. Once information is obtained, the student is required to analyze, determine relationships, and draw conclusions.

Inquiry is an integral part of certain clinical simulations that are used for teaching diagnostic and patient-handling skills. After a patient problem is presented, the student asks for information about the patient's appearance; requests results of laboratory tests, x-rays, and so forth; and can be provided with actual clinical data, such as breath sounds and heart sounds. A program of this type can be used for teaching and evaluating the process of making a medical or nursing diagnosis and selecting interventions.

The inquiry mode is also appropriate for use in research courses in which data needs to be manipulated and presented to students who then decide what conclusions can be drawn. Patterns of data can be altered to present various outcomes that require different conclusions. The student involved in either the clinical simulation or the research simulation has an opportunity to integrate knowledge and skills and apply acquired information to an actual problem situation, thus achieving a higher level of learning than would be possible in a nonparticipatory activity. Table 14-3 contains an example from a program in the inquiry mode.

Simulation. This section deals with the use of a computer for presenting and manipulating information about a model of a real-life situation or process. The reader is referred to Chapter 3 for the general discussion of purposes, process, and types of simulation.

In a computer simulation, the computer is used as the vehicle to present a model of a real-life situation, provide data requested by the student, incorporate the student's decisions into the system, and provide the student with feedback about effects of decisions made. The program is fully controlled by the student's questions and decisions, which are fed into the system. Once a decision is made, the computer responds with a new set of facts based on the consequences (both good and bad) of the decision. Thus, computer simulation is a dynamic process reflecting many successive decisions over a period of time. As with any simulation, computer simulation helps to deal with the constraints posed by clinical

Table 14-3
Excerpt from a Computer-Assisted Program Using Inquiry

```
MRS. S., A 32-YEAR-OLD BLACK WOMAN WHO IS
SEPARATED FROM HER HUSBAND, HAS BEEN REFERRED FOR
PSYCHIATRIC CONSULTATION FROM THE DERMATOLOGY
CLINIC.  YOU MAY MAKE FIVE SELECTIONS FROM THE
DATA MENU GIVEN TO GATHER DATA ABOUT THE PATIENT.
ONCE YOU HAVE RECEIVED THE DATA IN THE FIVE AREAS,
YOU WILL BE ASKED TO GIVE YOUR DIAGNOSTIC
IMPRESSION.

        1.   REASON FOR M.D. OR N.P. REFERRAL FROM THE
             CLINIC.
        2.   PATIENT'S VERSION OF REASON FOR REFERRAL.
        3.   FINDINGS AT THE REFERRING CLINIC.
        4.   HISTORY OF SIMILAR PROBLEMS.
        5.   PATIENT'S DESCRIPTION OF THE PROBLEM.

       10.   APPEARANCE AND BEHAVIOR DURING INTERVIEW.
       11.   MENTAL STATUS.

       21.   CRYING SPELLS.
       22.   SUICIDAL THOUGHTS OR ATTEMPTS.

TYPE IN THE NUMBER OF YOUR FIRST SELECTION AND
THEN HIT THE "RETURN" KEY.

1

THE PATIENT COMES TO THE CLINIC COMPLAINING OF
"BODY ODOR" BUT THERE ARE NO UNUSUAL ODORS
APPARENT TO THE EXAMINING NURSE PRACTITIONER.
NEXT SELECTION?

2

I HAVE HAD A STRANGE ODOR FOR A LONG TIME AND
MANY DOCTORS HAVE TOLD ME THAT IT'S "ALL IN MY
HEAD".  NEXT SELECTION?

5

I HAVE EXPERIMENTED WITH MYSELF TO SEE IF
DIFFERENCES IN WEIGHT OR HOW MUCH I SMOKE MAKES
ANY DIFFERENCE IN THE ODOR.  IT DOESN'T SEEM TO
MATTER, BUT I THINK THERE IS LESS ODOR WHEN I AM
AT EASE AND RELAXED.  NEXT SELECTION?

11
```

```
MRS. S. IS ALERT, ORIENTED, INTELLIGENT, AND HER
MEMORY APPEARS INTACT.  HER EMOTIONAL EXPRESSION
IS APPROPRIATE BUT VERY LIMITED AND FLAT.  THERE
IS NO EVIDENCE OF PERSECUTORY DELUSIONS OR
HALLUCINATIONS.  NEXT SELECTION?

21

MRS. S. REPORTS THAT SHE CRIES A LOT--SOMETIMES IN
PUBLIC.  SHE IS UNABLE TO SAY WHAT PRECIPITATES
THE TEARS.  YOU HAVE COMPLETED GATHERING DATA ON
THIS PATIENT.  IN YOUR OPINION, DOES MRS. S. HAVE
A PSYCHIATRIC PROBLEM?  TYPE YES OR NO.

yes

RIGHT.  WHICH DIAGNOSTIC CATEGORY DO YOU THINK
WOULD BE MOST LIKELY?  TYPE THE NUMBER OF THE
CATEGORY FROM THE LIST BELOW TO INDICATE YOUR
CHOICE.
```

SOURCE: University of California, San Francisco. Used by permission of Martin Kamp, M.D., Computer Center.

education—time, patient safety, and limited availability of desired experiences. The student is able to gain a sense of the total picture by participating in patient care from beginning to end. All students can be provided with the desired experiences without dependence on clinical availability. The student can experiment with various alternatives without fear of doing something wrong or causing harm to a patient.

The interaction between the student and the computer program in a computer simulation is illustrative of the inquiry mode previously discussed. The dialogue mode is also often a part of computer simulation, with the author of the program providing consultation, guidance, or criticism at designated times or when requested by the student. An added advantage is that, upon completion of the program, the computer can provide the student and/or the instructor with a summary or critique of the student's decisions and suggest remedial work when that is indicated.

Most computer simulations in medical and nursing education involve the simulation of patient care problems. Three basic types of patient models are used: the static patient, the dynamic patient, and the dynamic physiological system or disease process (Farquhar et al., 1978). In the static patient model the patient's condition does not change as a result of the interaction. The computer program simply provides information that is requested by the student and the student arrives at a conclusion based on the information obtained. In the dynamic patient model the program is capable of altering the patient's condition in response to student actions. The condition is then communicated to the student who uses the information to make subsequent decisions or requests for information. In the dynamic physiological system or disease process model there is a simulation of biological systems. This extends the dynamic patient model by providing data about common disease states in response to treatments and by demonstrating effects of drugs on physiological processes.

Holland and Hawkins (1972, p. 375) predicted that "simulation is likely to become one of the most widespread modes of instructional use (of the computer) in higher education." Although computer simulation has been used for a number of years in such areas as business administration, economics, and medical education, applications in nursing are limited. Several potential areas of use for the teaching or evaluating of clinical problem-solving skills exist, for example, basic nursing education, training of nurse practitioners, in-service education, continuing education, credit by examination and advanced placement of students, and relicensure or recertification (Table 14-4 is a sample computer program using simulation of a clinical problem-solving situation. Table 14-5 is an example of a simulated interview situation.)

Games. Both simulation games and nonsimulation games can be adapted for use with the computer. (The reader is referred to Chapter 3 for examples of simulation and nonsimulation games.) The gaming concept implies competition between two or more players (one of whom may be the computer program) to achieve a specific goal. In a computer game, the program is designed to assess strategies, give results or effects of decisions made, and introduce variables that alter the course of events.

The most common applications of computer games in higher education have been in business, economics, and management areas. No computer game applications to nursing have been found; however, many games that have been developed for noncomputer use could be readily adapted for use with a computer. In addition, games developed for other fields can be adapted for use in nursing education or used, as designed, for purposes that are common with those of other disciplines. As an example of the latter, Metro-Apex,* a computerized simulation game, is designed to give participants an understanding of health care systems (Washburn & McGinty, 1977). Participants receive feedback

*Available from the Center for Multidisciplinary Educational Exercises (COMEX), University of Southern California, Los Angeles, California 90007.

Table 14-4
Excerpt from a Computer-Assisted Program Using Simulation of a Clinical Problem-Solving Situation Plus Dialogue

```
YOU ARE ON DUTY IN THE EMERGENCY ROOM WHEN A
6-YEAR-OLD CHILD IS BROUGHT IN BY HIS PARENTS.
THE CHILD APPEARS ALERT BUT WEAK, DOES NOT ATTEMPT
TO STAND OR WALK, AND HIS SKIN IS PALE AND COOL.
THE FATHER TELLS YOU THAT HE THINKS THE CHILD
SWALLOWED SOME PILLS FROM THE MEDICINE CABINET.
HE FURTHER TELLS YOU THAT THE CHILD'S MOTHER HAS
'HEART TROUBLE' AND SUFFERS FROM 'FUNNY BEATS' AND
THAT THE CHILD'S OLDER SISTER IS EPILEPTIC AND
TAKES MEDICATION FOR SEIZURES.  WHEN THE CHILD WAS
FOUND, ALL THE DRUGS WERE MISSING.  THE FATHER
ASSUMES THAT THE CHILD EITHER SWALLOWED THEM OR
POURED THEM DOWN THE DRAIN.  NEITHER PARENT CAN
GIVE YOU ANY MORE INFORMATION ABOUT THE TYPE OR
QUANTITY OF DRUGS THAT HAD BEEN STORED IN THE
MEDICINE CABINET.  PLEASE HIT 'RETURN' WHEN YOU
ARE READY TO CONTINUE.

AT THIS POINT, THE CHILD BECOMES RESTLESS AND
VOMITS.  LOOKING AT THE VOMITUS CONFIRMS THAT
THERE IS NO RECOGNIZABLE DRUG TO BE SEEN.  WHAT
TEST OR PHYSICAL FINDING DO YOU WANT TO CHECK
FIRST?  TYPE YOUR ANSWER.

respiration

GOOD, MAKE SURE THE PATIENT IS BREATHING WELL.
SINCE THE CHILD HAS JUST VOMITED, YOU SHOULD CHECK
HIS RESPIRATION TO MAKE SURE HE HAS NOT ASPIRATED
ANY VOMITUS.  INITIAL DATA ABOUT THE PATIENT . . .
RESPIRATION IS 20 PER MINUTE AND AIRWAY IS CLEAR.
RADIAL PULSE IS INITIALLY IRREGULAR IN STRENGTH
AND RHYTHM, THEN REGULAR AT 80 PER MINUTE.
REMEMBER, YOU HAVE NO OTHER PHYSICAL DATA SO FAR.
WHAT TEST OR PHYSICAL FINDING DO YOU WANT NOW?
TYPE YOUR ANSWER.

electrocardiogram

YES, THE CARDIOGRAM IS A VERY GOOD CHOICE, BUT
DON'T FORGET TO CHECK THE BLOOD PRESSURE, WHICH IS
IMPORTANT AND CAN BE DONE VERY EASILY.  THE BP IS
110/70.  THE ECG (LEAD II) SHOWS A SERIES OF SINUS
BEATS, SEVERAL PVC'S, DEPRESSED S-T SEGMENTS, AND
SLIGHTLY PROLONGED P-R INTERVALS.  PLEASE HIT
"RETURN" WHEN YOU ARE READY TO CONTINUE.
```

223

```
THE CHILD HAS NO PRIOR HISTORY OF CARDIAC PROBLEM
AND WE MAY ASSUME THAT HIS ARRHYTHMIA RESULTED
FROM INGESTION OF TOXIC AMOUNTS OF A DRUG.  THE
DRUG INGESTION TOOK PLACE 3 HOURS AGO.  THE
PARENTS DID NOT NOTICE ANY SYMPTOMS AFTER THE
INGESTION OR UP UNTIL THE TIME THEY BROUGHT THE
CHILD TO THE HOSPITAL.  WHAT DRUG GROUP DO YOU
SUSPECT AS THE MOST LIKELY CAUSE OF THIS DRUG
TOXICITY?  TYPE THE DRUG NAME.

digitalis

VERY GOOD.  YOU CORRECTLY INTERPRETED THE
ARRHYTHMIA, THE ECG SIGNS, AND THE VOMITING AS
CLASSICAL SIGNS OF DIGITALIS POISONING.  DON'T
FORGET, HOWEVER, THAT OTHER DRUGS CAN CAUSE
ARRHYTHMIAS AND VOMITING, INCLUDING THE
ANTIARRHYTHMIC AGENTS.  PLEASE HIT 'RETURN' WHEN
YOU ARE READY TO CONTINUE.
```

SOURCE: University of California, San Francisco. Used by permission of Martin Kamp, M.D., Computer Center.

about effects of decisions on the community and health care system. Each round lasting 3 to 8 hours is equivalent to 1 year. Roles include elected officials, public health department officials, environmental personnel, hospital administrators, representatives of special interest groups, and others. Although no nurses are included, Metro-Apex offers potential advantages for use with any group, such as graduate students in community health nursing, who need to develop insight about interrelationships among elements of the health care system, interaction between the health care system and the larger community, and long term health care planning. Table 14-6 summarizes the purposes, goals, and points of control of the lesson with each of the six CAI types discussed.

Research Related to Effectiveness of CAI

Research about the effectiveness of using CAI in higher education settings is limited. The findings of a few studies in nursing and other fields at both the undergraduate and graduate levels are summarized here. Several conclusions based on the findings will be presented.

Three studies on the use of CAI at the undergraduate level for sub-

Table 14-5

Excerpt from a Computer-Assisted Program Using Simulation of an Interview
Situation

YOU ARE CONDUCTING THE INITIAL INTERVIEW WITH A
PSYCHIATRIC PATIENT. YOU MAY TALK TO THIS PATIENT
BY TYPING YOUR QUESTIONS AND RESPONSES OR BY NOT
TYPING ANYTHING IF YOU WANT TO RESPOND WITH
SILENCE. AFTER THE INTERVIEW IS COMPLETED, YOU
WILL BE ASKED WHETHER OR NOT YOU CARE TO MAKE A
DIAGNOSIS. HIT "RETURN" WHEN YOU ARE READY TO
CONTINUE.

THE PATIENT ENTERS YOUR OFFICE. YOU INTRODUCE
YOURSELF. HE IS SLENDER, CONVENTIONALLY DRESSED,
AND APPEARS TO BE ABOUT 30 YEARS OLD. YOU SEAT
YOURSELF AND ASK HIM TO BE SEATED. HE SITS DOWN
AND SAYS . . . THANK YOU.

what can I do for you, Mr. Sanders?

WELL, MY WIFE WANTED ME TO COME.

why did your wife want you to come?

IT'S NOT MY IDEA, THAT'S FOR SURE. MY WIFE JUST
TOLD ME I OUGHT TO SEE A PSYCHIATRIST. SHE SAID
SHE WAS GOING TO LEAVE IF I DIDN'T GO.

why do you think she said that?

I DON'T WANT TO TALK ABOUT MY WIFE.

(silence)

HOW COME YOU NEVER SAY ANYTHING, ANYWAY? THAT'S
WHAT I HEAR ABOUT YOU GUYS. YOU JUST SIT THERE
AND NEVER DO ANYTHING.

well, I need to know more about you.

I THOUGHT YOU WOULD WANT ME TO TELL YOU ALL ABOUT
MYSELF.

fine, start wherever you want.

WELL, I'M A PAINTER . . . NOT ONE OF THEM ARTISTS,
YOU KNOW . . . A HOUSEPAINTER. MAKE PRETTY GOOD
MONEY AT IT, TOO . . . AND BEEN WORKING PRETTY
STEADY.

I see

```
LATELY I'VE BEEN WORKING FOR THIS CONTRACTOR.
WE'RE ON AN APARTMENT JOB NOW.

(silence)

SAY, HOW COME YOU WANT TO KNOW SO MUCH ABOUT MY
JOB?

you can tell me about something else if you want.

YOU DON'T THINK THEY'LL FIND OUT AT WORK ABOUT ME
COMING HERE, DO YOU?

why, what if they did?
```

SOURCE: University of California, San Francisco. Used by permission of Martin Kamp, M.D., Computer Center.

Table 14-6
Summary of CAI Types, Purposes, Goals, and Point of Control of Lesson

CAI Type	Purpose	Goal	Control of Lesson
Tutorial	Presentation of new content	Acquisition of basic facts and concepts	Computer/author of program
Drill-and-Practice	Reinforcement and practice with previously learned content	Practice with material for fixing of concepts	Computer/author of program
Dialogue	Assistance and feedback to students during learning	Enrichment of the learning experience; increased student motivation and control	Student/learner
Inquiry	Presentation of situations/data from which students can draw conclusions	Enrichment; integration of knowledge and skills; independent decision making	Student/learner
Simulation	Presentation and manipulation of a model of real phenomena about which students can make decisions	Provide insight about actual situations; develop problem-solving skills; integration of knowledge and skills	Usually student/learner but can be combined
Game	Provide competitive situation in which outcome is defined	Development of insight into various strategies for reaching defined goal	Usually student/learner but can be combined

jects other than nursing present results about learning effectiveness, amount of time for learning, and attrition of students. They are:

1. Hansen, Dick, and Lippert (1968) found that there was no significant difference in test performance of students in a CAI physics course when compared with students in either a lecture course only or a lecture course plus review questions by computer. The most significant finding, however, was that the CAI group showed a time savings in learning of approximately 12 percent over the other groups.

2. Suppes and Jerman (1969) compared two groups of students studying elementary Russian. One group worked at a computer terminal for 50 minutes each day for the academic year while the control group received regular classroom instruction, attended a language laboratory, and submitted homework assignments. The students working with the computer performed at a significantly higher level. Perhaps of equal importance was the difference in dropout rate between the two groups: 30 percent for the computer-based section and 70 percent for the control group.

3. In an experimental multimedia gross anatomy course for freshmen (Jones et al., 1978), lectures were replaced by audiovisuals, CAI, and tutorial sessions. By looking at course exams, students in the experimental course were compared, over a period of 5 years, with the students in traditional courses. Out of 35 examinations (19 practical and 16 written), the experimental group performed significantly better six times (four practical and two written exams) while the traditional group performed significantly better three times (two practical and one written exam). Of particular interest are the records of average study times, which indicated that the students in the experimental group used, on the average, approximately one-third of the time required by the traditional group.

Three studies in undergraduate nursing education discuss learning effectiveness as the result of CAI using a system developed at the University of Illinois (see the discussion of PLATO later in this chapter). One of the studies also includes data about amount of time for learning. They are:

1. Bitzer (1966) compared the posttest scores of experimental and control groups in a diploma program during their study of the care of a patient with angina pectoris and myocardial infarction. The groups were matched in level of preinstruction knowledge. The experimental group received their instruction using the computer system ac-

companied by a short film of a typical patient case history. Traditional methods, including lectures, readings, case histories, and nursing care plans, were used with the control group. The results showed that the computer taught group scored significantly better than the control group on the posttest.

2. A later study in the same setting (Bitzer & Boudreaux, 1969) investigated the effectiveness of CAI for teaching maternity nursing. The students in one course were divided into two groups that, according to pretest results, were matched in their preinstruction level of knowledge about the topic. The control group was taught in the conventional classroom manner while the experimental group received instruction using the computer system. While posttest scores showed that students in both groups made a significant gain in learning, final examination results showed no significant difference between the two groups. However, the total time required by the students learning via computer ranged from 28 to 50 hours (including review time) while the control group spent 84 hours in the classroom.

3. Kirchhoff and Holzemer (1979), using a posttest only design without a control group, examined the effectiveness of using a CAI program for teaching students in a baccalaureate program about postoperative nursing care. It was their conclusion that the students learned the material.

Three studies in graduate or postgraduate education in nursing, medicine, and teacher training are summarized below:

1. Hoffer, Barnett, Mathewson, and Loughrey (1975) studied the application of CAI to instruction of hospital nurses in cardiopulmonary resuscitation. The results indicated that those nurses who used the computer increased their test scores in the cardiopulmonary resuscitation program while nurses in the control group using traditional in-service methods did not. They further demonstrated the importance of designing programs to meet the needs of a specific group since the nurses in this study objected to the use of criteria that clearly were developed for physicians.

2. Formal evaluation of the use of a computerized mannequin for training residents in anesthesiology was conducted using experimental and control groups (Holland & Hawkins, 1972). The results demonstrated that members of the experimental group achieved proficiency in less time and with fewer trials than that required by members of the group taught by traditional methods.

3. In a study of postgraduate teacher education using CAI transported

by truck to remote areas, Cartwright and Cartwright (1972) found CAI to be effective for training teachers in the field to recognize children with educational handicaps. CAI students were compared with students taking the same course by traditional lecture method in relation to time for completion of the course and performance on an identical final exam. Findings were that the CAI group scored 24 percent higher on the exam than did the control group and finished the course in a mean time of 25.2 hours in comparison to 37.5 hours for the non-CAI group. Operating costs for teaching the two groups were comparable.

Conclusions. The nine studies just cited seem to provide support to the following conclusions:

1. CAI is an effective learning technique. Students using CAI learn at least as well, and sometimes significantly better, than students using traditional classroom methods

2. CAI provides equivalent or greater learning in either the same amount or with significant savings of student time in comparison to learning by traditional methods.

3. CAI is cost-effective when the program is developed around specific objectives and educational needs.

4. The use of CAI can affect student attitudes and increase success, resulting in lower dropout rates.

These conclusions are comparable to those drawn by other authors reviewing research results in other areas (Bundy, 1971; Cross, 1976; Edwards et al., 1975; Jamison et al., 1974).

Values of Using Computers for Instruction

The values of CAI, regarding effectiveness, time-savings, and attitudes of students, have already been outlined in the research and conclusions cited above. However, some authors, both in general and nursing education, are of the opinion that the greatest potential strength of CAI is in its capacity to individualize instruction (Cross, 1976; Suppes, 1971; Magidson, 1977; Neher, 1975; Collart, 1973; Valish & Boyd, 1975; Porter, 1978; Reed et al., 1972).

The impact of computers on individualizing instruction can be great as they have the capacity to coordinate and present a wide range of stimuli as well as manage the instructional experience according to the needs of each individual student. Some specific ways that a computer can help to individualize instruction include:

1. Gives immediate feedback about performance
2. Makes adjustments in type and depth of content covered
3. Allows student control over time of study and pacing of lesson
4. Requires that the student actively participate in learning
5. Provides attention on a one-to-one basis
6. Provides data to the teacher and student about student progress and performance so that individualized assignments can be made
7. Allows the student the opportunity to experiment or be wrong without feeling embarrassed
8. Permits students to proceed through a lesson in a manner appropriate to their own styles of learning

Another value that is indirectly related to individualization is that of freeing the teacher from routine, repetitive tasks so that greater attention can be given to more individualized aspects of the learning situation. When the teacher does not have to (1) give lectures on material that is widely accepted and noncontroversial, (2) participate in clerical tasks associated with record keeping about student performance and progress, (3) produce alternate test forms, and (4) administer and grade tests, more time can be given to personal attention to students, answering questions, leading discussions, providing guidance, and increasing the depth of learning experiences (Bitzer & Boudreaux, 1969). Greater emphasis can be given to teaching and evaluating in the clinical setting. Thus, there is more effective (and challenging) use of both teacher and student time; the teacher's attention can be focused on those activities that are uniquely human; and students can be provided the help needed to make the learning experience more productive in relation to a higher level of curricular goals.

Another value that is unrelated to individualization, except in the sense of curriculum improvements, is the ability to obtain feedback about courses and lessons for serious evaluation of instruction. Precise data about both individual and group performances can be generated in minutes (Suppes, 1971). Data thus obtained can help the teacher to become aware of both the strengths and problems associated with CAI material. Programs can be revised to deal with any problems and improve the overall effectiveness of the material. When the emphasis is on mastery of objectives by all students, this type of activity is vital in providing instruction that, in fact, allows all students to achieve mastery.

Extent of Use of CAI in Higher Education

The case for learning effectiveness, higher instructional quality, and individualization has been made in the preceding sections. What, then, is the extent of use of CAI in higher educational settings? Although individual examples of use are available, data to provide a clear picture about extent of use are limited. Data that are available show that use varies with type of setting and subject area. In a 1968 study reported by Comstock (1972a), only 39 percent of colleges and universities reported the use of computers. Of these, Comstock estimated that only 30 percent of the computer use was for instructional purposes. It is not clear how much of this was instruction with a computer versus that about the computer. The patterns apparent from the data presented are as follows:

Computer use is general only among the larger schools and those granting the higher degrees.

Computer use tends to increase with degree level.

Computer use tends to increase with size of institution.

Computer use is greater among public than among private schools, (Comstock, 1972a, p. 145)

In a California survey (Comstock, 1972b), it was found that a majority of general institutions used the computer for instruction about the computer and computing, and 45 to 50 percent, respectively, used it for research applications and as a teacher's aid and problem-solving tool. On the other hand, only 37 percent made use of the computer for simulation, demonstrations, and games and 10 percent for presenting instruction directly to the student.

Other surveys also show limited use of the computer for instruction in both general and nursing education settings. Cross (1976) reported on a survey of community colleges, done in 1974, in which only 16 percent of the surveyed colleges reported the use of CAI. Levine and Wiener (1975) cite research indicating that only 7 percent of nursing schools used CAI, although 47.1 percent stated that CAI was being considered. In a 1976 survey of National League for Nursing accredited associate and baccalaureate degree nursing programs with an enrollment of 250 or more, only 14.6 percent of the respondents reported the use of CAI (Thompson, 1980). Lack of use in nursing programs is further supported by a recent survey by Knippers (1981), which demonstrated that CAI was the least used among self-instructional methods.

In contrast to other areas of study, certain specialized areas, such as medicine, have made greater use of computers for instruction. For example, Votaw and Farquhar (1978) report that by 1975 two-thirds of the medical schools in the U.S. made some instructional use of computers. It is not clear, however, what the extent of use was in individual schools.

It is clear that CAI is not widely used in higher education, especially in nursing education. If CAI is effective and has the power to individualize learning, what is it that impedes the widespread and immediate adoption of CAI methods?

Barriers to Adoption of CAI.   The answer to the question is no doubt complex and multifaceted. In relation to nursing education, Valish and Boyd (1975) stated an opinion of Jerome Lysaught that many basic nursing schools do not examine their curricula or teaching methods and go on with "business as usual" in spite of changing technology and demands for alternatives in procedures. In agreement with that opinion for education in general is a statement by Murphy (1977, p. 15), "The view that the computer is 'probably suitable for administrative work and not a valid instructional medium' is still the status quo."

Others have attempted to identify potential hindering factors to computer use for education in general (Comstock, 1972b; Levien, 1972; Levien & Mosmann, 1972a and b; Magidson, 1977; Morrisey, 1975; Suppes, 1971); education of health professionals (Brigham, 1978; Casberque, 1978; Doull & Walaszek, 1978; Winter, 1978); and nursing education (Collart, 1973; Frantz, 1976; Levine & Wiener, 1975; Porter, 1978). Four factors that seem particularly pertinent to nursing education are identified and discussed in this chapter:

1. Lack of compatibility of hardware and software.
2. Lack of appropriate software.
3. Resistance of faculty.
4. High costs.

Lack of compatibility of hardware and software.   Several computer languages, each with its own characteristics, limitations, and applications, are used to develop CAI materials. The language used tends to bind the user to one machine type. Companies can even change the language used for programming from one computer model to another. The result is that a program developed for one system cannot be used on other systems unless it is translated into compatible language. In addition, programs can be carried in various forms, for example, cassettes and disks, which are not usable on another system. These situations interfere with the sharing of materials, a condition that is an economic necessity for some institutions to use CAI.

Several things need to take place in order to achieve the compatibility that would allow broader dissemination of software. They incude (1) setting up a software format that would make programs usable with a variety of hardware systems (Brigham, 1978); (2) increasing the standardization of computer systems; (3) adopting a common language to be used within each discipline (Walters, 1978); and (4) establishing national networks for use by major disciplines. With continued progress in these areas, access to high quality materials developed by subject experts would be possible for a greater number of institutions at less cost.

Lack of appropriate software. A major obstacle to widespread CAI use is the limited availability of suitable software for educational purposes. The lack is related both to the problem of incompatibility just discussed and to production. Development of course materials simply has not kept up with advances in computer technology. Software that is available may not meet unique curricular needs. Some faculty may resist the use of materials developed by other people. Accessibility to programs via computer networks requires funds for initial hardware purchases, as well as the regular payment of user fees. In-house production is possible in some instances, but there are often problems since computers do not accept natural language programming, faculty do not have the required programming skills, or the incentives for faculty involvement with nontraditional strategies are lacking.

Certainly, increasing the compatibility of software with various systems and increasing the sharing among institutions could increase quality by allowing those who are experts to develop programs for widespread dissemination. With the emphasis placed on developing materials around broad concepts, programs would be more readily adaptable to an individual curriculum. Faculty who wish to become involved in the development of computer instructional programs need adequate support and assistance from programming and instructional design personnel. Quality should also increase as established publishers or specialized publishers of software enter the market, since competition will be greater and faculty will be more willing to develop materials that will be published.

Faculty resistance. The true potential for CAI cannot be realized without the support and involvement of faculty members. Faculty attitudes are thought to constitute one of the major barriers to the adoption of CAI. Resistance may be based on a variety of factors. One is that many faculty have had limited or no direct experience with computers and are intimidated by the technology they do not understand and the language they cannot use. Some do not know how to use CAI materials because the use of the computer as an instructional tool developed primarily in recent years. Even now most graduate programs do not include training in the use of CAI. Some faculty members feel threatened by technology that they fear could replace them. New methods that are thought to reduce one's own role in teaching may be resisted, especially by those who wish to keep the student in a dependent role.

Many, particularly young faculty members, hesitate to become involved in activities that do not carry the same incentives in the tenure/promotion process as those available through traditional research and publication. When materials are used only at the local level, they do not have the same value as materials that are published and widely distributed. Further, heavy teaching loads and related responsibilities, such as student advisement or committee work, may leave limited energy for the development of new materials and methods, especially when there is a lack of professional incentive.

Another element of faculty resistance may be based in the claim that CAI is impersonal and dehumanizing. Such an attitude may have developed as the result of administrative uses of the computer, personal experiences with computers in business settings, or the belief that any machine-based instruction is bad. Cross (1976) refers to several studies that fail to support the claim that CAI is impersonal and dehumanizing—at least from a student's perspective. Studies are available that show not only that student attitudes toward subject matter improve with CAI but also that some students, especially low achievers or those who do not respond well to conventional instruction, are especially enthusiastic about CAI. Others even view the computer as being "fairer" and more "likable" than the teacher.

Teachers must be convinced that computers will not replace them and that they can be allies in improving instruction. There need to be structured, positive experiences with CAI. Training sessions and workshops for teachers who have not had an opportunity to learn about CAI in their own graduate programs could help faculty members to develop skills in the facilitative role, become computer literate, and increase awareness of computer capabilities for helping them to improve teaching. Graduate programs preparing teachers need to increase their consideration of alternative strategies. Dedicated involvement of faculty is more likely to occur when participation results in recognition comparable to that of other efforts in research and publishing.

High costs.   The costs associated with purchase or leasing of hardware systems, membership in computer networks, and purchase or production of software makes it impossible for many institutions to participate in CAI without outside funding. Time-sharing and independent small systems have greatly reduced the costs; however, many educators and administrators are hesitant to invest in systems that may soon be modified or become obsolete, given recent technological advances, or that are incompatible with other systems. Costs of hardware are expected to continue to decrease while computing capabilities increase. In fact, Miller (1981) predicts that by 1985 a pocket computer with the power and speed of current large computers will be available at reasonable cost.

Related to cost is the expenditure in relation to instructional hours. True figures are difficult to discern since they are dependent on a number of factors—type of system, number of users, useful life of material, frequency of use, and cost of software purchase or production. Estimates of costs in several different settings and different programs are available (Doull & Walaszek, 1978; Kamp & Burnside, 1974; Zemper, 1978; Tidball, 1978; Starkweather & Kamp, 1978; Cross, 1976; Rau, 1977). The estimates provide support for the prediction that CAI can be competitive with conventional methods and may, in the future, cost much less than conventional methods. Costs are expected to continue to decrease with newer technology. Cost-effectiveness in fields that are considered to be more costly, such as nursing and medicine, may be easier to achieve than in other disciplines that do not require a clinical component.

So far, the decreasing hardware costs have not been accompanied by comparable reductions in cost of software. Some of this is due to inflation and the increasing complexity and sophistication of programs (Miller, 1981). Software costs are expected to be a critical factor in the future. Highly sophisticated programs that have a small user following are not economical. Although there has been little marketing activity for CAI materials at the university level (Bork, 1978), the demand for computer-based instructional materials may be similar to that which now exists for textbooks if the expected advances in the development of microcomputers occur (Winter, 1978). As publishers enter the software market, and if regional and national networks continue to develop, the costs will be spread over a greater number of users, resulting in lower costs for each individual user. As costs decrease, an individual with a microcomputer may be able to purchase or rent CAI software (Winter, 1978) or gain access via communication networks on a home television screen. The resulting possibilities for expansion of educational opportunities are obvious.

Examples of Applications to Nursing

Several examples of applications of CAI to nursing are evident in the literature. A few will be summarized here to give the reader an idea about what is available. Both individual applications and computer networks are included.

Individual Applications

The Ohio State University College of Medicine. The Ohio State University (OSU) College of Medicine is a leader in computer applications to health sciences education (Pengov, 1978). The OSU system is used primarily for undergraduate medical education, nursing education, allied health professions education, continuing health sciences education, and patient and nonmedical support staff education. Programs are used locally, regionally (see discussion of CAIREN later in this chapter), and nationally (see discussion of HEN later in this chapter). Many programs on a variety of medical topics are offered, with 51 programs indexed specifically for nursing education. The baccalaureate program in nursing at OSU requires eight of the programs to be completed by all students and designates seven others as optional. The programs utilize, primarily, the tutorial and dialogue modes with case studies (Hoye & Wang, 1973). Examples of programs available for nursing are (1) BOTTLE: Includes six modules on the topic of closed drainage systems of the chest for integration into a surgical nursing course (Collart, 1973; Hoye & Wang, 1973); (2) VEINS: Covers venipuncture and intravenous (IV) therapy in programs to fit several different educational levels of professional groups (Hoye & Wang, 1973; Winter, 1978); and (3) CCNUR: A three-part course, taking 5 to 7 hours to complete, that reviews cardiac anatomy and physiology and pathophysiology of heart disease for use by nurses preparing for work in coronary care units (Hoye & Wang, 1973).

Boston College. Boston College, Chestnut Hill, Massachusetts, uses computer simulations of patient assessment in the inquiry and dialogue modes for evaluation of clinical learning (Olivieri & Sweeney, 1980). The system used is a portable microcomputer and keyboard connected to an ordinary television set. Of particular interest is the economy of the system and the potential for using the programs on a home computer, if desired. Capabilities include audio recordings and the display of charts, graphs, and drawings on the television screen. Four programs are described involving a patient with a myocardial infarction being admitted to four settings: the emergency room, coronary care unit, general medical unit, and cardiac rehabilitation program after discharge. Users pose questions as they would in nursing assessment and the "patient" responds to the questions asked. The programs are designed to allow different levels of sophistication and include the opportunity to obtain laboratory results, vital signs, and ECG tracings. Sessions are accompanied by an evaluation test booklet, which the student completes and turns in to a teacher for evaluation.

The University of Michigan.   At the University of Michigan School of Nursing, a computer is used to respond to an epidemiology public health problem (Donabedian, 1976). The computer program allows students to check their own answers to a written exercise. The student interacts with the program regarding symptoms and possible causative organism of food poisoning. The series of questions is designed to reinforce basic epidemiological principles and tools, introduce simple statistics, and enhance intellectual skills in problem solving.

University of California, San Francisco.   Kamp and Burnside (1974) describe an experimental graduate psychiatric nursing class using CAI. The technique used was a simulated clinical situation with the computer program providing a brief patient description followed by the student asking a limited number of questions in order to collect further data and make a diagnosis. Program design was such that no important elements could be omitted. The computer program was followed by a theoretical discussion about content and interviewing techniques and an actual patient interview in the clinical setting. The results of the experimental course indicated that after using the computer program students were less anxious during actual clinical experience.

Pennsylvania State University, University Park.   Estes (1976) and Hall (1976) describe the use of CAI as part of an extended option, van-mounted system. Traditional paper-and-pencil "challenge" exams have been replaced by computer-managed self-study assessment in each of seven basic nursing courses. Registered nurses can obtain credit that is applied toward the baccalaureate degree in nursing.

Newman and O'Brien (1978) describe the use of computer-simulated research designs to provide graduate students with experience in the entire research process in a relatively short period of time without having to become directly involved in data collection. They use a data-generating computer program developed at the University of Michigan that allows progression from simple to complex designs using from one to multiple variables. Students are able to complete two experiments in 1 semester and test a proposed research design before actual implementa-

tion. A major learning benefit is increased understanding of interpreta-
tion of findings in relation to stated hypotheses.

Continuing education.   In addition to the use of CAI in basic instruction and evaluation, there are those who believe that CAI has great
potential in the continuing education of nurses (Meadows, 1977; Porter,
1978). CAI materials can be used (1) to provide basic instruction so that
staff development instructors can channel their efforts toward helping
to improve clinical judgment and competence (Reed et al., 1972); (2) for
verifying prior clinical knowledge in nursing (Valish & Boyd, 1975); and
(3) for continuing education of nurses in both hospital settings and
remote areas (Winter, 1978).

Computer Networks

Programmed Logic for Automated Teaching Operations (PLATO).   This system of CAI was initiated at the University of Illinois in 1960 and work in
nursing began in 1963 (Bitzer, 1966; Bitzer & Boudreaux, 1969; Hody
& Avner, 1978). In addition to investigating the role of the computer in
the instructional process, a major purpose was to develop hardware and
software that would be less costly than the nontechnical tools that were
replaced (Rockart & Morton, 1975). One result has been the development of an inexpensive visual display terminal, which is sensitive to
touch and has a projected cost of less than $500. Development of the
system has gone through several stages identified by Roman numerals,
that is, PLATO I, II, and so forth. The PLATO Health Sciences Network was established in 1974 (Bloomfield et al., 1978) and presently
consists of 50 systems across the United States (Winter, 1978).

Programs consist primarily of textual information and visual displays
and diagrams and use magnetic audio disks in the tutorial, inquiry, and
simulation modes. The system emphasizes quick access to audio and
visual materials by the use of magnetic audio disks and electronic slide
selectors. Programs on PLATO that are utilized in nursing include (1)
Maternity, a 12-unit course in maternity nursing (Bitzer & Boudreaux,
1969; Hoye & Wang, 1973); (2) *Care of the Patient with Angina Pectoris and
Myocardial Infarction,* a 90-minute session on this topic for use in a course
in medical-surgical nursing (Bitzer, 1966); and (3) *Pharmacology for
Nurses,* the mathematics of drugs and solutions, drug therapy, and drug
classifications (Hoye & Wang, 1973).

PLATO is also used in graduate nurse-midwifery programs (Nabor,
1975) and offers potential for improved administration and evaluation
of the Patient Management Problem (PMP) (Sherman et al., 1979).

Computer assisted simulation of the clinical encounter (CASE).   This is a model developed at the University of Illinois and refined at OSU (Pengov, 1978). Although intended for use in undergraduate medical education, it offers great potential for evaluation of clinical competence (Harless et al., 1978) and for use with any professional group needing practice in clinical decision making. With CASE the student assumes responsibility for a patient at the moment the patient seeks care and retains that responsibility until the medical problem is successfully, or unsuccessfully, resolved. Typically, the only unsolicited information received is an initial description of the patient and the setting. After that the student must type questions at the terminal in order to receive the information needed to make a diagnosis and plan treatment. The student "interviews" the patient to obtain medical and physical history data and obtains physical exam findings, laboratory data, and so forth, by requesting specifics desired. Additional data can be requested at any time. Once the student enters a diagnosis and treatment plan, feedback in the form of a description of the program author's diagnosis, suggested treatment, and listing of critical concepts is provided (see Pengov, 1978, pp. 274–276 for a sample CASE interaction).

Computer-Assisted Teaching System (CATS).   This system was developed by the Department of Pharmacology at the University of Kansas Medical Center in 1970 (Doull & Walaszek, 1978). In 1974, a consortium of 50 members in the United States and Europe was established. The programs are used by a variety of allied health fields, including undergraduate and graduate nursing students. The system includes both CMI and CAI components. CAI programs involve simulation with case studies as well as the tutorial mode with and without branching. Students at the University of Kansas have the option of using CAI materials, traditional methods, or a combination of the two. Although specific titles for nursing applications are not given, the units in a medical student pharmacology course include topics suitable for nurses: General Principles of Pharmacology, Autonomic Nervous System (ANS) and Cardiovascular Pharmacology, Central Nervous System (CNS) Pharmacology, and Chemotherapy and Blood Drugs.

The Computer Assisted Instruction Regional Education Network (CAIREN).
CAIREN is a regional network for sharing CAI learning resources at the Ohio State University College of Medicine with Ohio health care facilities and educational institutions (Forman et al., 1978). It became operational in 1969 with the principal purpose of providing relevant programs at accessible sites for continuing education and professional

growth of medical, nursing, and allied health personnel. Members include community hospitals, technical schools, and mental health institutions. Users include patients and families, clerical support personnel, and students and practicing professionals in medicine, nursing, and allied health. Several professional groups, including the Ohio State Nurses' Association, have approved selected programs for continuing education credit.

The Health Education Network (HEN).   This network was established in 1975 as an outgrowth of the Lister Hill National Center for Biomedical Communications Network, an experimental CAI network supported by the National Library of Medicine that existed from 1971 to 1975 (Tidball, 1978). The purpose of HEN is to "facilitate, maintain, and preserve economic, nationwide access to computer-assisted instructional materials for health education" (Tidball, 1978, p. 195). It is the first fully operational national network for the health sciences and provides access via terminals in numerous cities to the many programs available at Massachusetts General Hospital and the Ohio State University College of Medicine (see Tidball, 1978, p. 198). Computerized clinical case simulations are available on a 24-hour basis to member medical, nursing, and dental schools, hospitals, and health care institutions throughout the United States and Canada (Held & Kappelman, 1976), thus offering everexpanding prospects for both basic and continuing education in various health care fields.

FUTURE POSSIBILITIES

It is possible that in the future the computer will be a dominant force in higher education through its capacity to both individualize instruction and help students to learn how to learn (McKeachie, 1978). Major trends that are likely to affect the future of CAI relate to microprocessor and laser technology. Typical are the "fourth generation" computers, which are faster, smaller, cheaper, and have greater memory than their predecessors. The movement toward the use of simpler, natural languages is common. A characteristic in the future may be the ability to synthesize and recognize human speech. If this occurs, a user will be able to converse with a computer using natural language.

Laser technology has brought about the ability to store massive amounts of information on videodisks and holographic memory devices (Walters, 1978; Kahn, 1978; Kemph, 1981). The videodisk is inexpensive, durable, easily stored, and capable of incorporating all types of media—slides, motion, audio, print, and so forth. Holographic techniques make it possible to produce three-dimensional images at different magnifications. Both videodisk and holography have the capacity for high speed, random access of information at any desired point in a program and offer significant advantages for authoring of programs. Schneider (1975) believes that it is only a matter of time before videodisk replaces all conventional audiovisual media in educational institutions.

If current trends in decreasing costs and increasing portability and capability continue, and if problems related to compatibility, software production, and faculty resistance are effectively dealt with, the majority of students in higher educational settings should be deeply involved in CAI of all types by the year 2,000. Computer literacy will be a requirement for all undergraduate students. Terminals will be common in homes, as well as in schools. The student will be able to use a wide variety of well-developed, sophisticated programs using media of all types. Programs will be selected based on personal interests and learning styles. Software will be durable and easily transportable with many available for purchase or rental. Other programs will be accessible via satellite systems or telephone lines for display on home television screens. Programs will be available any time the student wishes to use them. Many will allow interaction with the student at a level close to that which occurs in direct teacher–student encounters. Students who are blind or deaf will be able to select the method of interaction suitable for them. The opportunity will exist for students to obtain degrees from universities that are far distant from where they live. Continuing education and professional development programs will be widely available. Grades will be either nonexistent or assigned solely on the performance of students in relation to specific, explicit criteria rather than in comparison to other students. Teachers' time will be used for development of quality instructional materials, diagnosis and management of the learning process, validation and evaluation of clinical learning and judgment, and interaction with individuals and small groups. Both the teacher and student will be able to obtain immediate data about student performance or a profile of the total educational experience that will be used in a nonpunitive way to plan learning experiences for students that will help them to achieve their educational/professional goals.

SUMMARY

Six types of CAI have been discussed in this chapter. Other areas discussed include research related to effectiveness of CAI, values of using

computers for instruction, and individual and computer network examples of application to nursing education. The computer is one of the
most significant, potentially revolutionary contributions of technology to
education. CAI is currently being used in some nursing education settings; however, the extent of use is limited, in spite of its ability to
individualize instruction, increase the quality of learning, and deal with
several constraints of clinical learning. Several factors that interfere with
the adoption and widespread use of CAI are identified. Should these
areas be adequately revolved, the potential for CAI in both basic and
continuing education in nursing is great.

References

Aavedal, M., Coombe, E., Fisher, C., Jones, M., & Standeven, M. Developing student–professor contracts in the clinical area. *International Nursing Review,* 1975, *22*(4), 105–108.

Abt, C. C. *Serious games.* New York: Viking Press, 1971.

Airasian, P. W. The role of evaluation in mastery learning. In J. H. Block (Ed.), *Mastery learning: Theory and practice.* New York: Holt, Rinehart & Winston, 1971.

Allen, D., & Ryan, K. *Microteaching.* Menlo Park, Calif.: Addison-Wesley, 1969.

Allen, R. M. Media and the University of Texas System School of Nursing. *Educational Resources & Techniques,* summer 1974, 9–12.

Anderson, H. E., White, W., & Wash, J. A. Generalized effects of praise and reproof. *Journal of Educational Psychology,* 1966, *57*(3), 169–173.

Anderson, R. H. Team teaching in the elementary and secondary schools. In A. de Grazia and D. Sohn (Eds.), *Revolution in teaching: New theory, technology, and curricula.* New York: Bantam Books, 1964.

Atwood, A. The mentor in clinical practice. *Nursing Outlook,* 1979, *27,* 714–717.

Ausubel, D. P. *The psychology of meaningful verbal learning: An introduction to school learning.* New York: Grune & Stratton, 1963.

The Bachelor of Science in Nursing, Statewide Nursing Program. Long Beach, Calif.: The Consortium of the California State University and Colleges, 1981. (Brochure)

Baker, E. H. A pre-Civil War simulation for teaching American History. In S. S. Boocock & E. O. Schild (Eds.), *Simulation games in learning.* Beverly Hills, Calif.: Sage, 1968.

Bales, R. F., & Slater, P. E. Role differentiation in small decision-making groups.

In T. Parsons and R. F. Bales (Eds.), *Family: Sociological and interaction process.* New York: The Free Press, 1955.

Barnard, J. D. The lecture-demonstration versus the problem-solving method of teaching a college science course. *Science Education,* 1942, *26,* 121–132.

Barrows, H. S. Simulated patients in medical teaching. *Canadian Medical Association Journal,* 1968, *98,* 676.

Barrows, H. S. *Simulated Pts (Programmed Pts): The development and use of a new technique in medical education.* Springfield, Ill.: Charles C. Thomas, 1971.

Barrows, H. S., & Abrahamson, S. The programmed patient: A technology for appraising student performance in clinical neurology. *Journal of Medical Education,* 1964, *39*(8), 802–805.

Belch, J. *Contemporary games* (Vol. 1). Detroit, Mich.: Gale Research Co., 1973.

Benner, P., & Benner, R. V. *The new nurse's work entry: A troubled sponsorship.* New York: Tiresias Press, 1979.

Berte, N. R. (Ed.) *Individualizing education through contract learning.* University, Ala.: The University of Alabama Press, 1975. (a)

Berte, N. R. The future for learning contracts. In N. R. Berte (Ed.), *Individualizing education through contract learning.* University, Ala.: The University of Alabama Press, 1975. (b)

Bevis, E. O. *Curriculum building in nursing* (2nd ed.). St. Louis: C. V. Mosby, 1978.

Beyers, M., Dickelmann, N., & Thompson, M. Developing a modular curriculum. *Nursing Outlook,* 1972, *20,* 643–647.

Bitzer, M. Clinical nursing instruction via the PLATO simulated laboratory. *Nursing Research,* 1966, *15*(2), 144–150.

Bitzer, M. D., & Boudreaux, M. C. Using a computer to teach nursing. *Nursing Forum,* 1969, *8*(3), 234–254.

Blair, M. G. How learning theory is related to curriculum organization. *Journal of Educational Psychology,* 1948, *29,* 161–166.

Blatchley, M. E., Herzog, P. M., & Russell, J. D. Effects of self-study on achievement in a medical-surgical nursing course. *Nursing Outlook,* 1978, *26,* 444–447.

Blechert, T., Torgrimson, S., & Schoeneberger, R. Auto-tutorial method for teaching manual skills. *American Journal of Occupational Therapy,* 1975, *29*(4), 219–221.

Bloom, B. S. *Taxonomy of educational objectives. Handbook I: Cognitive domain.* New York: David McKay, 1956.

Bloom, B. S. Learning for mastery. *Instruction and curriculum* (Topical papers and reprints No. 1). Durham, N.C., Regional Education Laboratory for the Carolinas and Virginia, 1968, 11 pp. (Mimeographed)

Bloom, B. S. The new direction in educational research: Alterable variables. *Phi Delta Kappan,* 1980, *61,* 382–385.

Bloom, B. S., Hastings, J. T., & Madaus, G. F. *Handbook on formative and summative evaluation of student learning.* New York: McGraw-Hill, 1971.

Bloomfield, D. K., Hody, G. L., & Levy, A. H. Some PLATO applications in health sciences education. In E. C. DeLand (Ed.), *Information technology in health science education.* New York: Plenum Press, 1978.

Boguslawski, M., & Judkins, B. Contemporary guidelines in teaching. *Journal of Nursing Education,* 1971, *10*(1), 3–11.

Boocock, S. S., & Schild, E. O. (Eds.) *Simulation games in learning.* Beverly Hills, Calif.: Sage, 1968.

Bork, A. Computers in the classroom. In O. Milton (Ed.), *On college teaching,* San Francisco: Jossey-Bass, 1978.

Bouchard, J., & Steels, M. Contract learning: The experience of two nursing schools. *Canadian Nurse,* 1980, *76*(1), 44–48.

Boyd, E. M. Contract learning. *Physical Therapy,* 1979, *59*(3), 278–281.

Bradley, A. P. Faculty roles in contract learning. In D. W. Vermilye (Ed.), *Learner-centered reform: Current issues in higher education, 1975.* San Francisco: Jossey-Bass, 1975.

Bradshaw, C. E. Concentrated experiential learning laboratories. *Journal of Nursing Education,* 1978, *17*(2), 32–35.

Brigham, C. R. Programming languages. In E. C. DeLand (Ed.), *Information technology in health science education.* New York: Plenum Press, 1978.

Brock, A. M. A study to determine the effectiveness of a learning activity package for the adult with diabetes mellitus. *Journal of Advanced Nursing,* 1978, *3,* 265–275.

Brodie, G. Reexamination of reinforcement in the learning process. *Journal of Nursing Education,* 1969, *8*(2), 27–30.

Broom, L., & Selznick, P. *Sociology.* Evanston, Ill.: Row, Peterson, 1958.

Brower, H. T. The external doctorate. *Nursing Outlook,* 1979, *27*(9), 594–599.

Bruner, J. *Toward a theory of instruction.* Cambridge, Mass.: Harvard University Press, 1966.

Bugelski, B. R. *The psychology of learning applied to teaching* (2nd ed.). Indianapolis: Bobbs-Merrill, 1971.

Bugelski, M. Technical aids to education. *Teaching Aid News,* 1964, *4*(14), 13–16.

Bundy, R. F. Computer-assisted instruction—where are we? In R. A. Weisgerber (Ed.), *Perspectives in individualized learning.* Itasca, Ill.: Peacock, 1971.

Burnside, I. M. Peer supervision: A method of teaching. *Journal of Nursing Education,* 1971, *10*(3), 15–22.

Burr, D. F. The schoolhouse of 1980. In J. E. Duane (Ed.), *Individualized instruction—programs and materials.* Englewood Cliffs, N.J.: Educational Technology Publications, 1973.

Cardarelli, S. M. The LAP—A feasible vehicle of individualization. *Educational Technology*, 1972, *12*(3), 23–29.

Carlson, E. *Learning through games.* Washington, D.C.: Public Affairs Press, 1969.

Carnegie Commission on Higher Education. *The fourth revolution: Instructional technology in higher education—A report and recommendations.* New York: McGraw-Hill, 1972.

Cartwright, G. P., & Cartwright, C. A. CAI course in the early identification of handicapped children. *Exceptional Children*, 1972, *38*, 453.

Casberque, J. Computer-assisted instruction in health professions education: Guidelines for utilization. In E. C. DeLand (Ed.), *Information technology in health science education.* New York: Plenum Press, 1978.

Chapman, J. J. Microteaching: How students learn group patient education skills. *Nurse Educator*, 1978, *3*(2), 13–16.

Cherryholmes, C. H. Some current research on effectiveness of educational simulations: Implications for alternative strategies. *American Behavioral Scientist*, 1966, *10*, 4–7.

Chickering, A. W. Developing intellectual competence at Empire State. In N. R. Berte (Ed.), *Individualizing education through contract learning.* University, Ala.: The University of Alabama Press, 1975.

Chinn, P., & Hunt, V. O. Teaching child nursing by modules. *Nursing Outlook*, 1975, *23*, 650–653.

Clark, C. C. Teaching nurses group concepts: Some issues and suggestions. *Nurse Educator*, 1978, *3*(1), 17–20.

Clark, T. F. Individualized education. In A. W. Chickering (Ed.), *The modern American college.* San Francisco: Jossey-Bass, 1981.

Coleman, J. S. The role of modern technology in relation to simulation and games for learning. In S. G. Tickton (Ed.), *To improve learning: An evaluation of instructional technology* (Vol. 1). New York: R. R. Bowker, 1970.

Collart, M. E. Computer assisted instruction and the teaching-learning process. *Nursing Outlook*, 1973, *21*, 527–532.

Collins, D. L., & Joel, L. A. The image of nursing is not changing. *Nursing Outlook*, 1971, *19*, 456–459.

Comstock, G. A. National utilization of computers. In R. E. Levien (Ed.), *The emerging technology: Instructional uses of the computer in higher education.* New York: McGraw-Hill, 1972. (a)

Comstock, G. A. The computer and higher education in California. In R. E. Levien (Ed.), *The emerging technology: Instructional uses of the computer in higher education.* New York: McGraw-Hill, 1972. (b)

Cooley, C. H. *Social organization.* New York: Scribner's, 1909.

Coombe, E. I., Jabbusch, B. J., Jones, M. C., Pesznecker, B. L., Ruff, C. M., & Young, K. J. An incremental approach to self-directed learning. *Journal of Nursing Education*, 1981, *20*(6), 30–35.

Cooper, S. S. Methods of teaching—revisited: Games and simulation, Part 8. *Journal of Continuing Education in Nursing,* 1979, *10*(5), 14; 47–48.

Cooper, S. S. Self-designed learning projects. In S. S. Cooper (Ed.), *Self-directed learning in nursing.* Wakefield, Mass.: Nursing Resources, 1980.

Covvey, H. D., & McAlister, N. H. *Computer consciousness: Surviving the automated 80's.* Menlo Park, Calif.: Addison-Wesley, 1980.

Cowart, M. E., & Burge, J. M. Evaluation by jury. *Nursing Outlook,* 1979, *27,* 329–333.

Craeger, J. G., & Murray, D. L. (Eds.) *The use of modules in college biology teaching.* Washington, D.C.: The Commission on Undergraduate Education in the Biological Sciences, 1971.

Craig, A. S. Contracting in a university without walls program. In N. R. Berte (Ed.), *Individualizing education through contract learning.* University, Ala.: The University of Alabama Press, 1975.

Craig, J. L., & Page, G. The questioning skills of nursing instructors. *Journal of Nursing Education,* 1981, *20*(5), 18–23.

Crancer, J., Maury-Hess, S., & Dunn, J. Contract systems and grading policies. *Journal of Nursing Education,* 1977, *16*(1), 29–35.

Crancer, J. A., & Maury-Hess, S. Games: An alternative to pedagogical instruction. *Journal of Nursing Education,* 1980, *19*(3), 45–52.

Cross, K. P. *Accent on learning.* San Francisco: Jossey-Bass, 1976.

Cruickshank, D. *The first book of games and simulations.* Belmont, Calif.: Wadsworth, 1977.

Cudney, S. A. Mediated self-instruction of basic nursing skills. *Nurse Educator,* 1976, *1*(2), 14–15.

Curtis, F. D., & Woods, G. G. A study of the relative teaching value of four common classroom practices in correcting examination papers. *School Review,* 1929, *37,* 616–623. Cited by N. M. Downie, *Fundamentals of measurement* (2nd ed.). New York: Oxford University Press, 1967.

Curtis, J., & Rothert, M. An instructional simulation system offering practice in assessment of patient needs. *Journal of Nursing Education,* 1972, *11*(1), 23–28.

Dale, A. G., & Klassen, C. R. *Business gaming: A survey of American collegiate schools of business.* Austin, Tex.: Bureau of Business Research, University of Texas, 1964.

Dale, E. *Audiovisual methods in teaching* (3rd ed.). New York: Holt, Rinehart & Winston, 1969.

Daniel, L., Eigsti, D., & McGuire, S. Teaching caseload management. *Nursing Outlook,* 1977, *25,* 27–29.

Dash, E. *Contract for grades.* Washington, D.C.: ERIC Clearinghouse on Higher Education, 1970.

Davidhizar, R. Use of simulation games in teaching psychiatric nursing. *Journal of Nursing Education,* 1977, *16*(5), 9–12.

Davis, G. L., & Eaton, S. L. On the move with microteaching. *American Journal of Nursing,* 1974, *74,* 1292–1293.

Dawson, M. D. Lectures versus problem-solving in teaching elementary soil sections. *Science Education,* 1956, *40,* 395–404.

Dearth, S., & McKenzie, L. Synoptics: A simulation game for health professional students. *Journal of Continuing Education in Nursing,* 1975, *6*(4), 28–31.

De Cecco, J. P. *The psychology of learning and instruction.* Englewood Cliffs, N.J.: Prentice-Hall, 1968.

De Cecco, J. P., & Crawford, W. R. *The psychology of learning and instruction* (2nd ed.). Englewood Cliffs, N.J.: Prentice-Hall, 1974.

Denson, J. S., & Abrahamson, S. Computer-controlled patient simulator. *Journal of the American Medical Association,* 1969, *208,* 504–508.

de Tornyay, R. Measuring problem-solving skills by means of the simulated clinical nursing problem test. *Journal of Nursing Education,* 1968, 7(3), 3–8; 34.

de Tornyay, R., & Searight, M. Micro-teaching in preparing faculty. *Nursing Outlook,* 1968, *16*(3), 34–35.

DeWalt, E. M., & Haines, A. K., Sr. The effects of specified stressors on healthy oral mucosa. *Nursing Research,* 1969, *18,* 22–27.

Dewey, E. *Dalton laboratory plan.* New York: E. P. Dutton, 1922.

Diamond, R. M. Piecing together the media selection jigsaw. *Audiovisual Instruction,* 1977, *22*(1), 50–52.

DiMinno, M., & Thompson, E. An interactional support group for graduate nursing students: A report. *Journal of Nursing Education,* 1980, *19*(3), 16–22.

Dirr, P. J. Is your media program only skin deep? *Audiovisual Instruction,* 1976, *21*(9), 24–26.

DiVesta, F. J. Instructor-centered and student-centered approaches in teaching a human relations course. *Journal of Applied Psychology,* 1954, *38,* 329–335.

Dollard, J., & Miller, N. E. *Personality and psychotherapy.* New York: McGraw-Hill, 1950.

Donabedian, D. Computer-taught epidemiology. *Nursing Outlook,* 1976, *24,* 749–751.

Dougan, M. A. Using "ICL" to meet the continuing learning needs of nurses . . . Individualized Contract Learning. *Journal of Continuing Education in Nursing,* 1980, *11*(1), 3–7.

Douglas, C. B. Making biology easier to understand. *The American Biology Teacher,* 1979, *41,* 277–299.

Doull, J., & Walaszek, E. J. The use of computer-assisted teaching systems (CATS) in pharmacology. In E. C. DeLand (Ed.), *Information technology in health science education.* New York: Plenum Press, 1978.

Dreher, R. E., & Beatty, W. H. *Instructional television project number 1: An experimental study of college instruction using broadcast television.* San Francisco: San Francisco State College, 1958.

Dreyfus, H. L., & Dreyfus, S. E. *The movement from novice to expert: What experience teaches.* Paper presented at the Achieving Methods of Intraprofessional Consensus Assessment and Evaluation Project Forum (Department of Health and Human Services, Public Health Services Grant #1 DIO NU 29024-03), San Francisco, 1981.

Duane, J. E. What's contained in an individualized instruction package. In J. E. Duane (Ed.), *Individualized instruction—programs and materials.* Englewood Cliffs, N.J.: Educational Technology Publications, 1973.

Dumke, G. S. *Authorization for implementation by the Consortium of a Statewide External Degree Program leading to the degree of Bachelor of Science in Nursing.* (Memorandum, Oct. 3, 1980)

Dunn, R., & Dunn, K. *Practical approaches to individualizing instruction: Contracts and other effective teaching strategies.* West Nyack, N.Y.: Parker, 1972.

Dunn, R., & Dunn, K. *Teaching students through their individual learning styles: A practical approach.* Reston, Va.: Reston, 1978.

Eaton, S., Davis, G. L., & Benner, P. E. Discussion stoppers in teaching. *Nursing Outlook,* 1977, *25,* 578–583.

Edwards, J., Norton, S., Taylor, S., Weiss, M., and Dusseldorp, R. How effective is CAI?: A review of the research. *Educational Leadership,* 1975, *33,*147–153.

Eggert, L. L. Challenge exam in interpersonal skills. *Nursing Outlook,* 1975, *23,* 707–710.

Ely, D., & Minars, E. The effects of a large scale mastery environment on students' self-concept. *Journal of Experimental Education,* 1973, *41*(4), 20–22.

Erickson, E. H., and Borgmeyer, V. Simulated decision-making experience via case analysis. *Journal of Nursing Administration,* 1979, *9*(5), 10–15.

Estes, C. A. *The use of computer based instruction in an extended degree program for nurses leading to the Bachelor of Science Degree.* Paper presented at the annual meeting of the American Educational Research Association, San Francisco, April 1976.

Eurich, A. C. A twenty-first-century look at higher education. In A. de Grazia and D. A. Sohn (Eds.), *Revolution in teaching: New theory, technology, and curricula.* New York: Bantam Books, 1964.

Farquhar, B. B., Hoffer, E. P., & Barnett, G. O. Patient simulations in clinical education. In E. C. DeLand (Ed.), *Information technology in health science education.* New York: Plenum Press, 1978.

Farran, D. C. Competition and learning for underachievers. In S. S. Boocock & E. O. Schild (Eds.), *Simulation games in learning.* Beverly Hills, Calif.: Sage, 1968.

Far Western Laboratory for Educational Research and Development. *Handbook for Minicourse III: Effective questioning in a classroom discussion.* Berkeley, Calif., 1969. (Mimeographed)

Feeney, J., & Riley, G. Learning contracts at New College, Sarasota. In N. R. Berte (Ed.), *Individualizing education through contract learning.* University, Ala.: University of Alabama Press, 1975.

Ferrell, B. Attitudes toward learning styles and self-direction of ADN students. *Journal of Nursing Education,* 1978, *17*(2), 19–22.

Flanagan, J. C. Individualizing education. In R. A. Weisgerber (Ed.), *Perspectives in individualized learning.* Itasca, Ill.: Peacock, 1971.

Foley, R. P., & Smilansky, J. *Teaching techniques: A handbook for health professionals.* New York: McGraw-Hill, 1980.

Forman, D. C., & Richardson, P. Open learning and guidelines for the design of instructional materials. *THE Journal, Technological Horizons in Education,* 1977, *4*(1), 9–12; 18.

Forman, M. H., Pengov, R. E., & Burson, J. L. CAIREN: A network for sharing health care learning resources with Ohio health care facilities and educational institutions. In E. C. DeLand (Ed.), *Information technology in health science education.* New York: Plenum Press, 1978.

Frantz, R. F. Computers in nursing education: Implications for the future. *Image,* 1976, *8,* 23–26.

Freeman, R. B., Croteau, L., & Lavoie, L. *Development of resources for independent and small group learning in a core curriculum.* Manchester, N.H.: Saint Anselm's College, 1975. (ERIC Document Reproduction Service No. ED 112938)

Gagné, R. M. *The conditions of learning.* New York: Holt, Rinehart & Winston, 1965.

Gagné, R. M., & Briggs, L. J. *Principles of instructional design.* New York: Holt, Rinehart & Winston, 1974.

Gall, M. D. The use of questions in teaching. *Review of Educational Research,* 1970, *40,* 707–721.

Gayles, A. R. Lecture vs. discussion. *Improving College and University Teaching,* 1966, *14,* 95–99.

Gibb, J. R. The effects of group size and of threat of reduction upon creativity in a problem-solving situation. *American Psychologist,* 1951, *6* 324. (Abstract)

Gibb, L. M., & Gibb, J. R. The effects of the use of "participative action" groups in a course in general psychology. *American Psychologist,* 1952, *7,* 247. (Abstract)

Gibbons, M. *Individualized instruction: A descriptive analysis.* New York: Teachers College Press, 1971.

Gillespie, J. The game doesn't end with winning. In S. Thiagarajan (Ed.), *Current trends in simulation/gaming.* Bloomington, Ind.: School of Education, Indiana University, 1973.

Glaser, R. *An individualized system*. Pittsburgh: University of Pittsburgh, Learning Research and Development Center, 1968. (Reprint #24)

Glaser, W. *Schools without failure*. New York: Harper & Row, 1969.

Glazier, R. *How to design educational games*. Cambridge, Mass.: Abt Associates, 1970.

Godejohn, C. J., Taylor, J., Muhlenkamp, A. F., & Blaesser, W. Effect of simulation gaming on attitudes toward mental illness. *Nursing Research*, 1975, *24*, 367–370.

Gordan, A. K. *Games for growth*. Palo Alto, Calif.: Science Research Associates, 1970.

Gudmundsen, A. Teaching psychomotor skills. *Journal of Nursing Education*, 1975, *14*(1), 23–27.

Guinée, K. K. *The aims and methods of nursing education*. New York: Macmillan, 1966.

Gustafson, M. B. Let's broaden our horizons about the use of contracts. *International Nursing Review*, 1977, *24*(1), 18–19; 24.

Hall, K. A. *The development and utilization of mobile CAI for the education of nurses in remote areas*. Paper presented at the annual meeting of the American Educational Research Association, San Francisco, April 1976.

Haney, J. B., & Ullmer, E. J. *Educational communications and technology* (2nd ed.). Dubuque, Ia.: Wm C Brown, 1975.

Hansen, D. N., Dick, W., & Lippert, H. T. *Research and implementation of collegiate instruction of physics via computer-assisted instruction*. Tallahassee: Florida State University, Nov. 1968. (Technical Report No. 3)

Hanson, K. H. Independent study: A student's view. *Nursing Outlook*, 1974, *22*, 329–330.

Harless, W. G., Farr, N. A., Zier, M. A., & Gamble, J. R. MERIT—an application of CASE. In E. C. DeLand (Ed.), *Information technology in health science education*. New York: Plenum Press, 1978.

Harms, M., & McDonald, F. J. A new curriculum design. *Nursing Outlook*, 1966, *14*(9), 50–53.

Held, T. H., & Kappelman, M. M. *Continuing education through computer technology*. Paper presented at the Health Education Medical Conference, Miami, Florida, 1976.

Herrscher, B., & Baker, G. A., III. *A systematic approach to instruction*. Durham, N.C.: Regional Educational Laboratory for Higher Education, 1969.

Hilgard, E. R. *Theories of learning* (2nd ed.). New York: Appleton-Century-Crofts, 1956.

Hoban, J. D. Successful simulations for health education. *Audiovisual Instruction*, 1978, *23*(9), 20–22.

Hoban, J. D., & Casberque, J. P. Simulation: A technique for instruction and evaluation. In C. W. Ford (Ed.), *Clinical education for the allied health professions*. St. Louis: Mosby, 1978.

Hody, G. L., & Avner, R. A. The PLATO system: An evaluative description. In E. C. DeLand (Ed.), *Information technology in health science education*. New York: Plenum Press, 1978.

Hoffer, E. P., Barnett, G. O., Mathewson, H. O., & Loughrey, A. Use of computer-aided instruction in graduate nursing education: A controlled trial. *Journal of Emergency Nursing*, 1975, *1*(2), 27–29.

Holland, W. B., & Hawkins, M. L. Technology of computer uses in instruction. In R. E. Levien (Ed.), *The emerging technology: Instructional uses of the computer in higher education*. New York: McGraw-Hill, 1972.

Holzemer, W. L., Schleutermann, J. A., Farrand, L. L., & Miller, A. A validation study: Simulations as a measure of nurse practitioners' problem-solving skills. *Nursing Research*, 1981, *30*, 139–144.

Honey, G. M. *Independent study project for seniors*. New York: National League for Nursing, 1975, 78–84. (NLN Publication No. 16–1538)

Hoose, D. C. A model for a nursing media center. *Nursing Outlook*, 1976, *24*, 104–106.

Horn, R. E., & Zuckerman, D. W. (Eds.) *The guide to simulation games for education and training*. Cranford, N.J.: Didactic Systems, 1977.

Horwitz, M. Hostility and its management in classroom groups. In W. W. Charters and N. L. Gage (Eds.), *Readings in the social psychology of education*. Boston: Allyn & Bacon, 1963.

Hovland, C. I. Computer simulation of thinking. In R. C. Anderson and D. P. Ausubel (Eds.), *Readings in the psychology of cognition*. New York: Holt, Rinehart & Winston, 1966.

Hoye, R. E., & Wang, A. C. (Eds.) *Index to computer based learning*. Englewood Cliffs, N.J.: Educational Technology Publications, 1973.

Hubbard, J. P., Levit, E. J., Schumacher, C. F., & Schnabel, T. G., Jr. An objective evaluation of clinical competence. *New England Journal of Medicine*, 1965, *272*, 1321–1328.

Huebner-Zappia, L. *Bibliography of games and simulations in health education*. Tucson, Ariz.: The University of Arizona, College of Education, Sim-Ed, Undated.

Humphrey, P. Learning about poverty and health. *Nursing Outlook*, 1974, *22*, 441–443.

Humphreys, L. G. Transfer of training in general education. *Journal of General Education*, 1951, *5*, 210–216.

Hunter, B., Kastner, C. S., Rubin, M. L., & Seidel, R. J. *Learning alternatives in U.S. education: Where student and computer meet*. Englewood Cliffs, N.J.: Educational Technology Publications, 1975.

Huntsman, A., & Thompson, M. A. Self-paced learning requires careful planning. *Cross-reference*, 1977, *7*(2), 1–3.

Hyman, R. Creativity and the prepared mind: The role of information and induced attitudes. In C. W. Taylor (Ed.), *Widening horizons in creativity.* New York: Wiley, 1964.

Infante, M. S. Toward effective and efficient use of the clinical laboratory. *Nurse Educator,* 1981, *6*(1), 16–19.

Ingalls, Z. Of cells, seeds, and students and the "Professor of the Year." *The Chronicle of Higher Education,* 1981, *22*(23), 5–6.

Interaction Associates. *Strategy notebook: Tools for change.* San Francisco: Interaction Associates, Inc., 1972.

Irby, D. M., & Morgan, M. K. (Eds.) *Clinical evaluations: Alternatives for health related educators.* Gainesville, Fla.: University of Florida, Center for Allied Health Instructional Personnel, 1974.

Ivor, F. A puzzling teaching method. *Journal of Continuing Education in Nursing,* 1974, *5*(6), 40–43.

Jackson, P. W. *The teacher and the machine.* Pittsburgh: University of Pittsburgh Press, 1966.

James, W. *Talks to teachers on psychology: And to students on some of life's problems.* New York: Holt, Rinehart & Winston, 1908.

Jamison, D., Suppes, P., & Wells, S. The effectiveness of alternative instructional media: A survey. *Review of Educational Research,* 1974, *44,* 1–67.

Jeffers, J. M., & Christensen, M. G. Using simulation to facilitate the acquisition of clinical observational skills. *Journal of Nursing Education,* 1979, *18*(6), 29–32.

Johnson, R. B., & Johnson, S. R. *Toward individualizing learning—A developers guide to self-instruction.* Menlo Park, Calif.: Addison-Wesley, 1975.

Johnson, W. D. *The effects of cognitive closure on learner achievement.* (Doctoral dissertation, Stanford University, 1965). (University Microfilms No. 65-2861).

Jones, A. L., & Kerwin, E. A guided independent study program for nurses. *Community College Frontiers,* 1978, *6*(2), 24–28.

Jones, N. A., Olafson, R. P., & Sutin, J. Evaluation of a gross anatomy program without dissection. *Journal of Medical Education,* 1978, *53,* 198–205.

Kagan, J., & Kogan, N. Individual variation in cognitive processes. In P. H. Mussan (Ed.), *Carmichael's manual of child psychology* (Vol. 1). New York: Wiley, 1970.

Kahn, G. S. Audiovisuals and computer-based learning. In E. C. DeLand (Ed.), *Information technology in health science education.* New York: Plenum Press, 1978.

Kamp, M., & Burnside, I. M. Computer-assisted learning in graduate psychiatric nursing. *Journal of Nursing Education,* 1974, *13*(4), 18–25.

Kaufmann, W. *The future of the humanities.* New York: Reader's Digest Press, 1977.

Keller, F. S., & Sherman, J. G. *The Keller plan handbook.* Menlo Park, Calif.: W. A. Benjamin, 1974.

Keller, M. L., & MacCormick, K. N. From graduate students to faculty: A simulation. *Nursing Outlook,* 1980, *28,* 305–307.

Keltner, J. W. *Group discussion processes.* New York: Green and Co., 1956.

Kemp, J. E. *Instructional Design* (2nd ed.). Belmont, Calif.: Fearon, 1977.

Kemph, J. Videodisc comes to school. *Educational Leadership,* 1981, *38,* 647–649.

Kirchhoff, K. T., & Holzemer, W. Student learning and a computer-assisted instructional program. *Journal of Nursing Education,* 1979, *18*(3), 22–30.

Knight, E. W. An improved plan of education, 1775. *School and Society,* 1949, *49*(1799), 409–411.

Knippers, A. *The use of self-instructional material in nurse education.* Unpublished doctoral dissertation, Indiana University, 1981.

Knowles, M. *The adult learner: A neglected species* (2nd ed.). Houston: Gulf Publishing, 1978.

Kolb, D. A. *The learning style inventory: Technical manual.* Newton, Mass.: Institute for Development Research, 1976.

Kolb, D. A., Rubin, I., & McIntyre, J. *Organizational psychology: An experimental approach.* Englewood Cliffs, N.J.: Prentice-Hall, 1971.

Koop, V. *The relationship of internal-external control and adjustment and satisfaction in structured and unstructured academic programs.* Waterloo, Ontario: Waterloo University Press, 1968, 1–44.

Kramer, M. Team teaching is more than team planning. *Nursing Outlook,* 1968, *16*(7), 47–48.

Kramer, M., Tegan, E., & Knauber, J. The effect of presets on creative problem solving. *Nursing Research,* 1970, *19,* 303–310.

Langford, T. Self-directed learning. *Nursing Outlook,* 1972, *20,* 648–651.

Langford, T. Establishing a nursing contract. *Nursing Outlook,* 1978, *26,* 386–388.

Laszlo, S. S., & McKenzie, J. L. The use of a simulation game in training hospital staff about patient rights. *Journal of Continuing Education in Nursing,* 1979, *10*(5), 30; 35–36.

Layton, J. Students select their own grades. *Nursing Outlook,* 1972, *20,* 327–329.

Layton, J. Instructional packaging. *Journal of Nursing Education,* 1975, *14*(4), 26–30.

Leavitt, H. J. Some effects of certain communication patterns on group performance. *Journal of Abnormal Social Psychology,* 1951, *46,* 38–50.

Lehmann, T. Evaluating contract learning. In D. W. Vermilye (Ed.), *Learner-centered reform: Current issues in higher education 1975.* San Francisco: Jossey-Bass, 1975.

Lenburg, C. B. The external degree in nursing: The promise fulfilled. *Nursing Outlook,* 1976, *24,* 422–428.

Leveck, P. An extended master's degree program. *Nursing Outlook,* 1975, *23,* 646–649.

Levien, R. E. Attitudes. In R. E. Levien (Ed.), *The emerging technology: Instructional uses of the computer in higher education.* New York: McGraw-Hill, 1972.

Levien, R. E., & Mosmann, C. Institutions. In R. E. Levien (Ed.), *The emerging technology: Instructional uses of the computer in higher education.* New York: McGraw-Hill, 1972. (a)

Levien, R. E., & Mosmann, C. Instructional uses of computers. In R. E. Levien (Ed.), *The emerging technology: Instructional uses of the computer in higher education.* New York: McGraw-Hill, 1972. (b)

Levine, D., & Wiener, E. Let the computer teach it. *American Journal of Nursing,* 1975, *75,* 1300–1302.

Lewis, D. R., Wentworth, D., Reinke, R., & Becker, W., Jr. *Educational games and simulations in economics.* New York: Joint Council on Economic Education, 1974.

Lewis, E. P. Secure in her skills. *Nursing Outlook,* 1971, *19,* 519.

Lewis, J. *Administering the individualized instruction program.* West Nyack, N.Y.: Parker, 1971.

Lincoln, R., Layton, J., & Holdman, H. Using simulated patients to teach assessment. *Nursing Outlook,* 1978, *26,* 316–320.

Lindquist, J. Strategies for contract learning. In D. W. Vermilye (Ed.), *Learner-centered reform: Current issues in higher education 1975.* San Francisco: Jossey-Bass, 1975.

Luchins, A. S. Mechanization in problem solving: The effect of "Einstellung." *Psychological Monographs,* 1942, No. 248.

Lyle, E. An exploration in the teaching of critical thinking in general psychology. *Journal of Educational Research,* 1958, *52,* 129–133.

Maatsch, J. L., & Gordan, J. J. Simulations in clinical evaluations. In D. M. Irby & M. K. Morgan (Eds.), *Evaluating clinical competence in the health professions.* St. Louis: Mosby, 1978.

Mager, R. F. *Preparing instructional objectives.* Palo Alto, Calif.: Fearon, 1962.

Mager, R. F. *Developing attitude toward learning.* Palo Alto, Calif.: Fearon, 1968.

Magidson, E. M. Is your module good? How do you know? *Audiovisual Instruction,* 1976, *21*(8), 43–44.

Magidson, E. M. One more time: CAI is not dehumanizing. *Audiovisual Instruction,* 1977, *22*(8), 20–21.

Markle, S. Teaching conceptual networks. *Journal of Instructional Development,* 1977, *1*(1), 13–17.

Marriner, A. Student self-evaluation and the contracted grade. *Nursing Forum,* 1974, *13,* 130–135.

Martens, K. H. Self-directed learning: An option for nursing education. *Nursing Outlook,* 1981, *29,* 472–477.

McBeath, R., McNall, L., Picker, R., Watts, T., Howard, T., Leveille, D., Provost, D. H., & Smart, J. M. *Self-paced learning: A perspective for those who seek to be innovative within the California State University and Colleges.* Los Angeles: Office of the Chancellor, Committee for New Program Development and Evaluation, 1974. (Mimeographed)

McDonald, R. L., & Dodge, R. A. Audio-tutorial packages at Columbia Junior College. In J. G. Craeger & D. L. Murray (Eds.), *The use of modules in college biology teaching.* Washington, D.C.: The Commission on Undergraduate Education in the Biological Sciences, 1971.

McGill, C., & Molinaro, L. Setting up and operating outreach centers for continuing education in nursing. *Journal of Continuing Education in Nursing,* 1978, *9*(1), 14–18.

McGuire, C., & Babbott, D. Simulation techniques in the measurement of problem-solving skills. *Journal of Educational Measurement,* 1967, *4,* 1–10.

McIntyre, H. M., McDonald, F. J., Bailey, J., & Claus, K. K. A simulated clinical nursing test. *Nursing Research,* 1972, *21,* 429–435.

McKay, S. R. A peer group counseling model in nursing education. *Journal of Nursing Education,* 1980, *19*(3), 4–10.

McKeachie, W. J. Research on teaching at the college and university level. In N. L. Gage (Ed.), *Handbook of research on teaching.* Chicago: Rand McNally, 1963.

McKeachie, W. J. Procedures and techniques of teaching: A survey of experimental studies. In N. Sanford (Ed.), *The American college.* New York: Wiley, 1966.

McKeachie, W. J. *Teaching tips: A guidebook for the beginning college teacher* (7th ed.). Lexington, Mass.: Heath, 1978.

McKenzie, L. Simulation games and adult education. *Adult Leadership,* 1974, *22,* 293–295.

McLuhan, M., & Fiore, Q. *The medium is the massage.* New York: Bantam Books, 1967.

Meadows, L. S. Nursing education in crisis: A computer alternative. *Journal of Nursing Education,* 1977, *16*(5), 13–21.

Memmer, M. K. Television replay: A tool for students to learn to evaluate their own proficiency in using sterile technique. *Journal of Nursing Education,* 1979, *18*(8), 35–42.

Miller, S. Technology: The future is now. *Black Enterprise,* June 1981, 58–62.

Milner, S. D. How to make the right decisions about microcomputers. *Instructional Innovator,* 1980, *25*(6), 12–19.

Milton, O. *Alternatives to the traditional.* San Francisco: Jossey-Bass, 1975.

Milton, O. (Ed.). *On college teaching.* San Francisco: Jossey-Bass, 1978.

Montag, M. *The education of nursing technicians.* New York: Putnam, 1951.

Moran, V. Facilitating self-directed learning: The role of the staff development director. In S. S. Cooper (Ed.), *Self-directed learning in nursing.* Wakefield, Mass.: Nursing Resources, 1980.

Morrisey, C. A. Electronic publishing in instruction. *THE Journal, Technological Horizons in Education,* 1975, *2*(8), 13–16; 32.

Murphy, T. M. Exorcising the ghosts in computing or C.A.I.: An applications approach. *THE Journal, Technological Horizons in Education,* 1977, *4*(5), 15; 18–20.

Nabor, S. Creative approaches to nurse–midwifery education. *Journal of Nurse–Midwifery,* 1975, *20*(3), 26–28.

Neher, W. R. A plea for productive dialogue in the design of computer based education. *THE Journal, Technological Horizons in Education,* 1975, *2*(2), 10–13; 22–23.

Newman, M. A., & O'Brien, R. A. Experiencing the research process via computer simulation. *Image,* 1978, *10,* 5–9.

Novak, J. *The future of modular instruction.* Ithaca, N.Y.: Cornell University, Center for Improvement of Undergraduate Education, 1973. (CIUE Notes No. 6)

O'Connell, A. L., & Bates, B. The case method in nurse practitioner education. *Nursing Outlook,* 1976, *24,* 243–246.

O'Connor, M. E., & Jones, D. An innovative teaching strategy for nursing education. *Journal of Nursing Education,* 1975, *14*(4), 9–15.

Olivieri, P., & Sweeney, M. A. Evaluation of clinical learning: By computer. *Nurse Educator,* 1980, *5*(4), 26–31.

Osborn, W. P. Dogmatism, tolerance for cognitive inconsistency, and persuasibility under three conditions of message involvement. *Proceedings of the 81st Annual Convention of the American Psychological Association,* 1973, *8,* 363–364. (Summary)

Osborn, W. P., & Thompson, M. A. Variables associated with student mastery of learning modules. In M. V. Batey (Ed.), *Communicating nursing research* (Vol. 9). Boulder, Colo.: Western Interstate Commission for Higher Education, 1977, 167–179.

Paduano, M. A. Introducing independent study into the nursing curriculum. *Journal of Nursing Education,* 1979, *18*(4), 34–37.

Page, G. G., & Saunders, P. Written simulation in nursing. *Journal of Nursing Education,* 1978, *17*(4), 28–32.

Paynich, M. L. Why do basic nursing students work in nursing? *Nursing Outlook,* 1971, *19,* 242–245.

Pearson, B. D. Simulation techniques for nursing education. *International Nursing Review,* 1975, *22,* 144–146.

Pengov, R. E. The evolution and use of computer-assisted instruction (CAI) in health sciences education at the Ohio State University College of Medicine. In E. C. DeLand (Ed.), *Information technology in health science education.* New York: Plenum Press, 1978.

Penta, F. B., & Kofman, S. The effectiveness of simulation devices in teaching selected skills of physical diagnosis. *Journal of Medical Education,* 1973, *48,* 442–445.

Phillips, G. M. *Communication and the small group* (2nd ed.). New York: Bobbs-Merrill, 1973.

Pipes, L. Getting started with microcomputers. *Instructional Innovator*, 1980, *25*(6), 10–11.

Porter, S. F. Application of computer-assisted instruction to continuing education in nursing: A review of the literature. *Journal of Continuing Education in Nursing*, 1978, *9*(6), 5–9.

Postlethwait, S. N., & Russell, J. D. Minicourses—the style of the future? In J. G. Craeger & D. L. Murray (Eds.), *The use of modules in college biology teaching*. Washington, D.C.: The Commission on Undergraduate Education in the Biological Sciences, 1971.

Price, A. W. The effective use of the multimedia approach in staff development. *Journal of Nursing Administration*, 1971, *1*(4), 38–45.

Price, G. E., Dunn, R., & Dunn, K. Productivity environmental preference survey. Lawrence, Kan.: Price Systems, 1979. (PEPS Manual)

Pullan, B., & Plant, S. M. Spot on!—that's the name of the game. *Nursing Mirror*, 1978, *147*(23), 26–29.

Raser, J. R. *Simulation and Society*. Boston: Allyn & Bacon, 1969.

Rau, J. L., Jr. Computer-assisted instruction: A solid-state Socrates? *Respiratory Care*, 1977, *22*, 581–593.

Rauen, K., & Waring, B. The teaching contract. *Nursing Outlook*, 1972, *20*, 594–596.

Raven, B. H., & French, R. P. Group support, legitimate power, and social influence. *Journal of Personality*, 1958, *26*, 400–409.

Ray, G. J., & Clark, C. E. The creation and use of an autotutorial learning system in a baccalaureate program in nursing. *THE Journal, Technological Horizons in Education*, 1977, *4*(6), 32–34; 47–48.

Reed, F. C., Collart, M. E., & Ertel, P. Y. Computer assisted instruction for continued learning. *American Journal of Nursing*, 1972, *72*, 2035–2039.

Reed, S. The overhead projector and transparencies. *Journal of Nursing Education*, 1968, *7*(2), 9–14.

Reinhart, E. Independent study: An option in continuing education. *Journal of Continuing Education in Nursing*, 1977, *8*(1), 38–42.

Reiser, R. A. Increasing the instructional effectiveness of simulation games. *Instructional Innovator*, 1981, *26*(3), 36–37.

Richards, A., Jones, A., Nichols, K., Richardson, F., Riley, B., & Swinson, R. Videotape as an evaluation tool. *Nursing Outlook*, 1981, *29*, 35–38.

Richardson, A. *Mental imagery*. New York: Springer, 1969.

Robinson, J. A. Simulation and games. In P. H. Rossi & B. J. Biddle (Eds.), *The new media and education*. Chicago: Aldine, 1966.

Rochin, M., & Thompson, M. A. Strategies for independent learning in nursing. *THE Journal, Technological Horizons in Education*, 1975, *2*(4), 15; 18–21.

Rockart, J. F., & Morton, M. S. S. *Computers and the learning process in higher education*. New York: McGraw-Hill, 1975.

Rockler, M. J. Applying simulation/gaming. In O. Milton (Ed.), *On college teaching*. San Francisco: Jossey-Bass, 1978.

Rogers, C. *Client-centered therapy: Its current practice, implications, and theory*. Boston: Houghton-Mifflin, 1951.

Rogers, C. *Freedom to learn*. Columbus, Oh.: Merrill, 1969.

Rogers, S. Testing the R. N. student's skills. *Nursing Outlook*, 1976, *24*, 446–449.

Rose, J., & Riegert, E. *Looking at the instructional developer from the client's point of view*. Paper presented at the annual meeting of the Association for Educational Communications and Technology, Anaheim, Calif., March–April, 1976.

Rose, T. L., Koorland, E. I., & Reid, B. Improving practicum performance: The CASE contract. *Contemporary Education*, 1978, *50*, 18–23.

Rossi, P. H., & Biddle, B. J. (Eds.) *The new media and education*. Chicago: Aldine, 1966.

Rottet, S. Gaming as a learning strategy. *Journal of Continuing Education in Nursing*, 1974, *5*(6), 22–25.

Russell, J. D. *Modular instruction* Minneapolis: Burgess, 1974.

Rynerson, B. C. Using videotapes to teach therapeutic interaction. *Nurse Educator*, 1980, *5*(5), 10–11.

Satterfield, J. Lecturing. In O. Milton (Ed.), *On college teaching*. San Francisco: Jossey-Bass, 1978.

Saupe, J. L. Learning and the evaluation process. In P. L. Dressel (Ed.), *Evaluation in higher education*. Boston: Houghton-Mifflin, 1961.

Schmidt, M. C. A self-paced ICU core curriculum. *Cross-reference*, 1977, *7*(2), 4–5.

Schneider, E. W. *Applications of videodisc technology to individualized instruction*. Paper presented at the National Science Foundation Conference for Ten Year Forecast for Computers and Communications, Warrenton, Va., September 1975. (ERIC Document Reproduction Service No. ED 158 722)

Scholdra, J., & Quiring, J. The level of questions posed by nursing educators. *Journal of Nursing Education*, 1973, *12*(1), 15–20.

Schweer, J. *Creative teaching in clinical nursing*. St. Louis: Mosby, 1972.

Secord, P. F., & Backman, C. W. *Social psychology*. San Francisco: McGraw-Hill, 1964.

Seidl, A. H., & Dresen, S. Gaming: A strategy to teach conflict resolution. *Journal of Nursing Education*, 1978, *17*(5), 21–28.

Shaffer, M. K., & Pfeiffer, I. L. Videotape as a method for staff development of nurses. *Journal of Continuing Education in Nursing*, 1978, *9*(6), 19–24.

Shaffer, M. K., & Pfeiffer, I. L. You too can prepare videotapes for instruction. *Journal of Nursing Education*, 1980, *19*(3), 23–27.

Shaftel, F., & Shaftel, G. *Roleplaying for social values: Decision-making in the social studies*. Englewood Cliffs, N.J.: Prentice-Hall, 1967.

Sherer, B. K., & Thompson, M. A. The process of developing a learning center in an acute care setting. *The Journal of Continuing Education in Nursing*, 1978, *9*(1), 36–44.

Sheridan, A., & Smith, R. A. Student-family contracts. *Nursing Outlook*, 1975, *23*, 114–117.

Sherman, J. E., Miller, A. G., Farrand, L. L., & Holzemer, W. L. A simulated patient encounter for the family nurse practitioner. *Journal of Nursing Education*, 1979, *18*(5), 5–15.

Shockley, J. A multi-faceted program for continuing education in nursing. *Journal of Nursing Education*, 1981, *20*(3), 20–26.

Shute, J. *Mastery learning and modules*. New York: National League for Nursing, 1976, 32–38. (NLN Publication No. 23-1618)

Siegel, L., & Siegel, L. C. The instructional Gestalt. In L. Siegel (Ed.), *Instruction: Some contemporary viewpoints*. San Francisco: Chandler, 1967.

Sim-Ed. *Catalog of educational simulations*. Tucson: The University of Arizona, College of Education, Sim-Ed, 1978.

Simpson, E. J. The classification of educational objectives. *Illinois Teacher of Home Economics*, 1966, *10*(1), 135–140.

Skinner, B. F. *Science and human behavior*. New York: Macmillan, 1953.

Skinner, B. F. *The technology of teaching*. New York: Appleton-Century-Crofts, 1968.

Slavin, R. E. Classroom reward structure: An analytical and practical review. *Review of Educational Research*, 1977, *17*, 633–650.

Slavin, R. E., & Tanner, A. M. Effects of cooperative reward structures and individual accountability on productivity and learning. *Journal of Educational Research*, 1979, *72*, 284–298.

Sloan, M. R., & Schommer, B. T. The process of contracting in community nursing. In B. W. Spradley, *Contemporary community nursing*. Boston: Little, Brown, 1975.

Smith, C. M. Learning on your own for credit. *American Journal of Nursing*, 1980, *80*, 2013–2015.

Solomon, R. L. Punishment. *American Psychologist*, 1964, *19*, 239–253.

Sommerfeld, D. P., & Hughes, J. R. How independent should independent learning be? *Nursing Outlook*, 1980, *28*, 416–420.

Sorensen, G. An honors program in nursing. *Nursing Outlook*, 1968, *16*(5), 59–61.

Sparks, S. M., & Mitchell, G. E. The National Medical Audiovisual Center. *Journal of Nursing Education*, 1978, *17*(1), 29–34.

Stanford Teacher Education Program. *Micro-teaching: A description*. Stanford, Calif.: Stanford University, 1967. (Mimeographed)

Starkweather, J. A., & Kamp, M. A self-contained CAI machine for health sciences education. In E. C. DeLand (Ed.), *Information technology in health science education*. New York: Plenum Press, 1978.

Stein, R. F., Steele, L., Fuller, M., & Langhoff, H. F. A multimedia independent approach. *Nursing Research,* 1972, *21,* 436–447.

Steiner, M. J., & Rothenberg, S. Teaching home health care with videotapes. *Nurse Educator,* 1980, *5*(4), 5–7.

Stonewater, J. K. A process model for simulation design. *Audiovisual Instruction,* 1978, *23*(5), 21–23.

Stuck, D. L., & Manatt, R. P. A comparison of audiotutorial and lecture methods of teaching. *Journal of Educational Research,* 1970, *63*(9), 414–418.

Sullivan, H. J., Schutz, R. E., & Baker, R. L. Effects of systematic variations in reinforcement contingencies on learner performance. *American Educational Research Journal,* 1971, *8,* 135–142.

Sullivan, K., Gruis, M., & Poole, C. From learning modules to clinical practice. *Nursing Outlook,* 1977, *25,* 319–321.

Suppes, P. Computer technology and the future of education. In R. A. Weisgerber (Ed.), *Perspectives in individualized learning.* Itasca, Ill.: Peacock, 1971.

Suppes, P., & Jerman, M. Computer-assisted instruction at Stanford. *Educational Technology,* 1969, *9*(1), 22–24.

Swendsen, L., Meleis, A., & Hourigan, J. Processes and strategies for implementation of learning modules in a nursing curriculum. *The Journal of Biocommunication,* 1977, *4*(2), 10–14.

Sylvester, M. J. Management games: A useful link between theory and practice. *Journal of Nursing Administration,* 1974, *4*(4), 28–32.

Taba, H. *Handbook for elementary social studies.* Palo Alto, Calif.: Addison-Wesley, 1967.

Tansey, P. J., & Unwin, D. *Simulation and gaming in education.* Toronto: Methuen Educational, Ltd., 1969.

Tarpey, K. S., & Chen, S-P. Team teaching: Is it for you? *Journal of Nursing Education,* 1978, *17*(2), 36–39.

Thiagarajan, S. *Experiential learning packages.* Englewood Cliffs, N.J.: Educational Technology Publications, 1980.

Thiagarajan, S., & Stolovich, H. *Instructional simulation games.* Englewood Cliffs, N.J.: Educational Technology Publications, 1978.

Thibaut, J. W., & Kelley, H. H. *The social psychology of groups.* New York: Wiley, 1959.

Thompson, M. Learning: A comparison of traditional and autotutorial methods. *Nursing Research,* 1972, *21*(5), 453–457.

Thompson, M. A. A systematic approach to module development. *Journal of Nursing Education,* 1978, *17*(8), 20–26.

Thompson, M. A. Status of innovative programs in nursing education—a survey. *Proceedings and Evaluation of the Learning Resources Center Conference,* Bethesda, Md., U.S. Dept. of Health and Human Services, 1980, *1,* 86–91.

Thorman, J. H., & Knutson, P. The option of retaking exams. *THE Journal, Technological Horizons in Education,* 1977, *4*(7), 43.

Thorndike, E. L. *Animal intelligence.* New York: Macmillan, 1911.

Tidball, C. S. Health Education Network. In E. C. DeLand (Ed.), *Information technology in health science education.* New York: Plenum Press, 1978.

Tosti, D. T., & Addison, R. A taxonomy of educational reinforcement. *Educational Technology,* 1979, *14*(9), 24–25.

Tough, A. M. *The adults learning projects.* Toronto: The Ontario Institute for Studies in Education, 1971. (Educational Research Series No. 3)

Tough, A. M. Interests of adult learners. In A. W. Chickering (Ed.), *The modern American college.* San Francisco: Jossey-Bass, 1981.

Trautman, P. *An investigation of the relationship between selected instructional techniques and identified cognitive style.* Unpublished doctoral dissertation, St. John's University, 1979.

Tuckman, B., Henkelman, J., O'Shaughnessy, P., & Cole, M. *The induction and transfer of search sets.* Paper presented at the meeting of the American Education Research Association, New York, February 1967.

Ubben, G. C. The role of the learning package in an individualized instruction program. *Journal of Secondary Education,* 1971, *46,* 206–209.

Valadez, A. M., & Heusinkveld, K. B. Teaching nursing students to teach patients. *Journal of Nursing Education,* 1977, *16*(4), 10–14.

Valish, A. U., & Boyd, N. J. The role of computer assisted instruction in continuing education of registered nurses: An experimental study. *Journal of Continuing Education in Nursing,* 1975, *6*(1), 13–32.

Verplanck, W. S. The control of the content of conversation: Reinforcement of statements of opinion. *Journal of Abnormal and Social Psychology,* 1955, *51,* 668–676.

Votaw, R. G., & Farquhar, B. B. Current trends in computer-based education in medicine. *Educational Technology,* 1978, *18*(4), 54–56.

Wales, S. K., & Hageman, V. Guided design systems approach in nursing education. *Journal of Nursing Education,* 1979, *18*(3), 38–45.

Walters, R. F. Planning for educational communication networks. In E. C. DeLand (Ed.), *Information technology in health science education.* New York: Plenum Press, 1978.

Ward, P. S., & Williams, E. C. *Learning packets: New approach to individualizing instruction.* West Nyack, N.Y.: Parker, 1976.

Washburn, A. W., & McGinty, R. T. The use of Metro-Apex in health administration and planning education and training. *Health Education Monographs,* 1977, *5* (Suppl. 1), 36–41.

Weisgerber, R. A. Individualized learning through technology. *Audiovisual Instruction,* 1973, *18*(3), 54–55.

White, D. T., & Lee, A. S. A baccalaureate nursing program satellite. *Nursing Outlook,* 1977, *25,* 394–398.

Wilson, S. R., & Tosti, D. T. *Learning is getting easier: A guidebook to individualized education.* San Rafael, Calif.: Individual Learning Systems, Inc., 1972.

Wing, R. L. Two computer-based economics games for sixth graders. In S. S. Boocock & E. O. Schild (Eds.), *Simulation games in learning.* Beverly Hills, Calif.: Sage, 1968.

Winter, J. M. Computer-assisted instruction in the continuing education of health professionals. *Journal of Allied Health,* 1978, 7, 206–213.

Witkin, H. A. *The role of cognitive style in academic performance and in teacher–student relations.* Princeton, N.J.: Educational Testing Service, 1973.

Witkin, H. A., & Moore, C. A. *Cognitive style and the teaching–learning process.* Paper presented at the annual meeting of the American Educational Research Association, Chicago, April 1974.

Wittkopf, B. Self-instruction for student learning. *American Journal of Nursing,* 1972, 72, 2032–2034.

Wolf, M. S., & Duffy, M. E. *Simulation/games: A teaching strategy for nursing education.* New York: National League for Nursing, 1979. (NLN Publication No. 23-1756)

Worby, D. Independent learning: The uses of the contract in an English program. *Lifelong Learning: The Adult Years,* 1979, 2(6), 32–34; 42.

Zemper, E. D. CAI at the Michigan State University Medical Schools. In F. G. DeLand (Ed.), *Information technology in health science education.* New York: Plenum Press, 1978.

Zides, E. Videocassettes at the Boston University School of Nursing. *Videoplay Magazine,* July 1974, 25–28.

Index